Music for Life

Aspects of Creative Music Therapy with Adult Clients

Music for Life Compact disc
Gary Ansdell
ISBN 1 85302 300 0

of related interest

Music Therapy in Health and Education
Edited by Margaret Heal and Tony Wigram
ISBN 1 85302 175 X

Music and People with Developmental Disabilities
Music Therapy, Remedial Music Making and Musical Activities
F W Schalkwijk
ISBN 1 85302 226 8

Making Music with the Young Child with Special Needs
A Guide for Parents
Elaine Streeter
ISBN 1 85302 187 3

Arts Therapies and Clients with Eating Disorders
Fragile Board
Edited by Ditty Dokter
ISBN 1 85302 256 X

Music for Life
Aspects of Creative Music Therapy with Adult Clients

Gary Ansdell

Jessica Kingsley Publishers
London and Bristol, Pennsylvania

First published in the United Kingdom in 1995 by
Jessica Kingsley Publishers Ltd
116 Pentonville Road
London N1 9JB, England
and
1900 Frost Road, Suite 101
Bristol, PA 19007, U S A

Library of Congress Cataloging in Publication Data
A CIP catalogue record for this book is available from the Library of Congress

British Library Cataloguing in Publication Data
A CIP catalogue record for this book is available from the British Library

ISBN 1-85302-299-3

Printed and Bound in Great Britain by
Cromwell Press, Melksham, Wiltshire

Contents

Part Three: Understanding the Creative Music Therapy Process

Music does not represent life: it *is* life

Charles Ives

The ultimate authority, however, remains the music itself. Whatever is said in this book will be proved right or wrong not by agreement or disagreement with one theory or another but by agreement or disagreement with the facts of the musical experience.

Victor Zuckerkandl: 'The Sense of Music'

in memory of Jo

Preface

'Words don't work: that's why we need music' wrote Anthony Burgess. An odd remark for a novelist perhaps, albeit one who composed music as a hobby. Many people, however, would echo something of his sentiment: that music gives them an experience they cannot put into words, or that they need music when words do not work. Music therapy, one of the newest incarnations of the art of music, rests on these facts.

Yet any book on music therapy faces head-on the paradox of using words to describe events and experiences which happened in music. This is even more so for the present book, where the main argument concerns the essential difference between musical and verbal processes (and consequently musical and verbal therapies). The accompanying CD is therefore not just an optional extra but part of the argument – the reader can also be a listener and hear, I hope, what sometimes only the music can convey.

My main aim for *Music for Life* was to describe how Creative Music Therapy,[1] an approach mostly known for its work with children, has been successfully used with adult clients in the last twenty years or so. The meat of the book is the selection of case studies I have collected from my own practice and from colleagues in England and Germany. These attempt to show the diversity of the work in this approach, one of whose strengths lies in the range of people for whom it can be appropriate and effective. Therapists currently work with adults living with mental health problems, learning difficulties and chronic illness; in prisons, hospitals, hospices and specialist settings such as the London Lighthouse (a centre for people living with HIV and AIDS).

---

1 I use 'Creative Music Therapy' as an alternative to 'Nordoff–Robbins Music Therapy' – an approach largely associated with work with children (see Introduction). Creative Music Therapy indicates an approach to music therapy with adult clients developed from the principles of Nordoff and Robbins' work.

Writing the case studies it became clear, however, that what I wanted to stress was not just the diversity of the work, but the essential similarity of principle which underpinned this diversity. There are indeed more similarities than differences in a music therapy session with an autistic child and one with a professionally trained musician. We work in much the same way with both people, and I hope that what comes through the case studies is how it is the principle of working through the music which remains the constant.

With the case studies as the meat of this book's sandwich structure, a second set of interleaving chapters reflect on themes emerging from the cases. These short essays concern aspects of the process of Creative Music Therapy such as creating, listening, expressing and meeting in the music: also how the phenomenon of music works in itself within music therapy to quicken people into action, connect them into a group or recall them into integration.

It has been characteristic of Creative Music Therapy that it does not rest on a single over-arching and extra-musical theory. Equally, I do not intend that the essay chapters in *Music for Life* add up to a complete theory of Creative Music Therapy with adult clients. Instead they gather together various relevant material from different literatures (philosophical, psychological and musicological) as reflections on, rather than theories of, aspects of the music-therapeutic process.

The insights from a musicological perspective are, I feel, especially important – for it is a central theme of this book that music therapy works in the way music works. We have to look at what is unique to music in order to find out what is unique to music therapy. Whether this can ever amount to a theory is perhaps dubious. As Peter Kivy (1993) has pointed out, what is often called 'music theory' is not theory in the sense of explanation, but rather a very detailed description of musical events. Given that music therapy rests on the facts of the musical experience it is likely that we should be equally suspicious of final theories of music therapy.

I found, additionally, that in order to make clear what Creative Music Therapy is, it became necessary also to say what it is *not*: to contrast it to some extent with other approaches to music therapy and to general assumptions of what we do.[2] I try to explain why Creative Music Therapy is not a form of psychotherapy, a 'New Age' technique, or music teaching.

The degree of confusion was illustrated in an article in *The Times* in 1992, when the reporter accused music therapists of 'playing different tunes'.

2 Readers wanting a survey of current approaches to music therapy are recommended: L. Bunt (1994) *Music Therapy: An Art Beyond Words* and K. Bruscia (1991) *Case Studies in Music Therapy*.

Though further proof of the rising profile of music therapy this also demonstrated the need for the various branches of the profession to clarify the differences as well as the commonalities of a wide-ranging discipline. To appropriate Adam Phillips' remark about psychoanalysis, music therapy can indeed be a circus with many acts. Yet with music therapy now in its late adolescence/early adulthood, it is perhaps no bad time to ask some leading questions – as a spur to further clarification and development. 'The search for identity, rather than the identical, can make for some interesting problems in music theory' wrote Thomas Clifton (1975). As is often the case, we can substitute 'music therapy' for 'music' with no loss of meaning.

I am grateful to Jessica Kingsley Publishers for agreeing to publish this book with the CD. Understanding the approach of Creative Music Therapy is greatly helped by being able to hear examples of the work.

There are many other people to thank – above all, the clients who have allowed us to write their stories and reproduce their comments and music; then, my colleagues Cheow Godfrey, Dagmar Gustorff, Peter Hoffmann, Colin Lee, Lutz Neugebauer and Rachel Verney for trusting me with their case studies and favourite musical excerpts. From the beginning it was decided that, rather than each therapist writing their own case study, I would collect them by interview and write them in my own style. These were then returned and re-written until the therapists were satisfied. I hope that I have done justice to their work and that something of their individuality still comes through. This book began as a joint venture between Rachel Verney and myself. Unfortunately two births and an emigration frustrated the project. I want to thank her, nevertheless, for her continued enthusiasm and support. Susanna Watson and David Aldridge were invaluable in their readings of the material, combining criticism and encouragement in just the right creative balance. Thanks also to Simon Woods for helping with the CD and Richard Egarr for setting up the musical examples. Finally the writing was made possible by the generous assistance of the Speedwell Trust and the John Stevens Trust.

A few years ago I attended a conference called 'Music for Life' on different forms of musical help for people with terminal illness. Music therapist Colin Lee (who has also contributed a case to this book) presented the work he had done over a period of three years with Francis, who had just died of AIDS. Francis had trained as a pianist, and their improvisations together were often of symphonic proportions. Colin went into no great explanations or interpretations but simply played long excerpts of the music they improvised together, along with some comments Francis had written about his experience of the music therapy process. The large audience at the conference were neither all music therapists nor indeed musicians. They simply listened spellbound to the sheer power of the music and to the relationship between these two people within it. The final excerpt he played was from what they knew was to be their last session together. The music was a slowly decreasing pulse of octaves extinguishing like a heart-beat. Suddenly it stopped and four hundred people collectively held their breath. The music had explained itself. It had also seemed somehow not just music played and listened to: but music *lived.*

Gary Ansdell
Institut für Musiktherapie, Herdecke
July 1994.

Part One

What is Creative Music Therapy?

Introduction

MUSIC, THERAPY AND MUSIC THERAPY

'What exactly are we doing here?' asked a client recently at the beginning of a first session – adding helpfully, 'I don't expect an answer!...but, I mean, are we just making music?' Though at the time I took the invitation not to give a long explanation, much of this book is an attempt to give him an answer and to explain, moreover, how this answer can be both 'yes' and 'no'.

An outside observer of our session may well have concluded that we were indeed 'just making music' – remarking that two people were both playing instruments and seemed to be communicating, even enjoying themselves. Were our observer, however, to ask both players *why* they were there, then she would find out something more: that the context and the expectations of the music-making were not the conventional ones of our society. Indeed, rather than the players describing themselves just as musicians who enjoyed playing together, one referred to himself as a 'therapist', the other as a 'client'.

Adult clients usually come to a music therapist (or are referred) because of a belief that music therapy involves something more than making music. Yet even the title of the profession can lead to confusions.'Music therapy' is both alike and unlike other helping professions such as physiotherapy, speech therapy or psychotherapy. With each of these it is clear where the therapeutic effort is directed: to the speech, body or (admittedly not so comfortably) the psyche. Music therapy is, however, clearly a different case. Quite simply, how does the music relate to the therapy?

Almost every music therapist would deny that their aim is, like the music teacher's, to improve the client's music. Many would, in fact, see this to be the last thing they do – that the music in music therapy is, on the contrary, a means to a non-musical end which is in many ways similar to that of the psychotherapist. In what has evolved as a 'music psychotherapy' the music is seen as facilitating words, and it is at this locus where the 'real' therapy is seen to be done.

A 'music psychotherapy' can thus be seen as one way of accommodating a therapeutic dimension within music therapy. Many music therapists, however, would maintain that this is not the only option – that it is indeed possible to have a 'purely musical' music therapy, where the therapeutic locus is still *within* the musical. The tradition of Creative Music Therapy has attempted to demonstrate the validity of this way of working: both with children and with adult clients who are verbally competent.

Stemming from this issue, two basic questions run through this book, as indeed they do through the whole of the current debate in music therapy: what is the relationship between music and therapy in music therapy? and, what is the relationship between music and words within the therapeutic process?

CREATIVE MUSIC THERAPY

Benjamin Britten wrote the Preface to a small book by Paul Nordoff and Clive Robbins called *Therapy in Music for Handicapped Children* (1971). Britten remarked that, at a time when the arts in general seemed to be losing their need to communicate, here was a musical approach 'where the concentration is entirely on just this, on communication pure and simple'.

Paul Nordoff was an American pianist and composer, Clive Robbins a teacher in special education. They met in England at a Sunfield Home for handicapped children, where they began a way of working in music using improvisation as a basis. During the next fifteen years, until Nordoff's death in 1976, they developed and taught this approach in Europe and America.[1]

Nordoff and Robbins worked initially with mentally handicapped, autistic and psychotic children, many of whom were cut off from verbal communication. They found, however, that music could be a powerful alternative when the children were actively and creatively involved in the process of music-making through improvisation. Nordoff and Robbins described their work not as music in therapy, but *therapy in music.* It was the music itself that reached the child directly and which formed the basis of a meeting between

1 They wrote a detailed book on the method called *Creative Music Therapy* (Nordoff and Robbins 1977). Since Paul Nordoff's death Clive Robbins has continued to practise, teach and promote the work along with a growing number of music therapists trained at institutes set up in London, Germany and New York.

the two people. This could then expand into a musical dialogue which could form the basis of a long-term therapeutic relationship.

In the last twenty years or so therapists trained to work with children in this approach have also begun to work with adult clients: initially those living with mental health problems or physical or mental handicaps, but increasingly with non-impaired clients with chronic illness, psycho-social and communication problems. The transition between working with children and adult clients was less problematic than may be imagined, largely because the underlying principle remains constant and effective whether the client is a handicapped child or a trained musician: namely that Creative Music Therapy works in the way music itself works, and that its 'results' are essentially of the same kind as music achieves for all of us. What I hope comes out of the case studies in this book is a demonstration of the power of music itself; how it can act within a person and how a therapeutic relationship with a person based on a purely musical relationship can be significant and transforming.

EXPLAINING MUSIC THERAPY

Creative Music Therapy is primarily a practical approach. Most therapists would rather have it seen as a special form of music-making than a musical form of clinical therapy, answerable to another system. The insights of Creative Music Therapy come largely from the experience of making music with a wide variety of people in different situations and with different needs.

Yet such statements must be considered alongside Even Ruud's comment that 'the field of music therapy can never establish theories and procedures separated from those within the field of psychology and philosophy' (Ruud 1980). We are back again to the subject of my client's question: whether, that is, there is a theory *behind* the obvious practical focus of the work. Is it possible to have a music therapy based on a 'mostly musical' model rather than one underpinned by an extra-musical treatment theory? If so, how is it possible to explain the method, aims and results behind such work to a client, referring doctor or funding agency?

The undeniable fact of music therapy's precarious balance between the world of music and the world of therapy has meant that various attempts have been made to ally some of its procedures, aims and explanatory models to those of prevailing treatment theories. Ruud (1980) identifies four main areas: physiological/'medical model', psychoanalytical, behavioural and humanistic/existential. Creative Music Therapy is no exception to theoretical influence, despite its basic musical orientation. Both anthroposophy and the tradition of humanistic psychology have influenced how the music–therapy equation is understood.

Yet there is a difference between, on the one hand acknowledging the influence of the ideas and values of other treatment theories and, on the other, having a music therapy explaining itself exclusively in terms of the concepts of another system, be this psychodynamic theory or anthroposophy. The danger is always that the focus of attention moves away from the musical component of the therapy and on to the conceptual system of whatever approach is being used.

An alternative option in explaining what happens in music therapy is to turn to a musicological model to help understand the purely musical aspects of the work. Here the specific structural components can be investigated – how, that is, a piece of music therapy (preserved on a tape) makes sense as a piece of music in its own right. The problem this time is that in converting the improvisation into an object (a transcribed score) a vital aspect of the music therapy process is lost – the way in which a client can be heard directly in the therapy room (or possibly on tape) with his or her living qualities.

In short, we find ourselves in a situation where an extra-musical theory tends to delete the 'object' (the music), whilst a musicological one deletes the 'subject' (the player or listener). For our hybrid discipline of music therapy we perhaps also need a hybrid understanding unique to the discipline. As Lesley Bunt (1994) has recently written, 'We could begin to develop a perspective from within the evolving discipline of music therapy itself... Perhaps by a deeper understanding of music and musical processes we shall begin to become aware once again of the central position of music within music therapy.' *Music for Life* attempts to demonstrate the possibility and validity of such a view. Working with adult clients in Creative Music Therapy has meant that, unlike the children Nordoff and Robbins worked with, they can report their experience and give us new insights into the varieties of musical and music-therapeutic experience.

The first part of this book begins with two chapters attempting to clarify the two parts of the hybrid: music and therapy. Chapter 1 looks at music not as an objective, historical entity but as something living and related to us: how its elements and structures relate to our bodies, thoughts and feelings and to our patterns of communication with other people. The second chapter, 'Therapy in Art' attempts to show how music and the other creative arts can work in a therapeutic context (but one not necessarily defined by a psychotherapeutic model). I finish Part One with a chapter based on a question-and-answer format, containing some of the commonest issues that come up in relation to music therapy in general and to Creative Music Therapy in particular.

CHAPTER 1

Becoming Music

> Many, if not all, of music's essential processes can be found in the constitution of the human body and its patterns of interaction with other bodies in society. (John Blacking)

It would be unusual for most books on music to begin with questions about the nature of music itself. The fundamentals of the medium are generally taken as given. A book about music therapy, however, needs to look again at just this level: at music as a phenomenon, and at how the basic 'ingredients' of musical experience can be made accessible to people in music therapy.

How does music relate to us as human beings? This is the question which any investigation in music therapy needs to start from. Indeed, what music therapy so powerfully demonstrates is the need for a more inclusive view of music: one, in short, which includes *us* in its explanations.

THE MUSIC WITHIN US

Let us start with some suggested definitions of music itself. That offered by the nineteenth-century critic Eduard Hanslick, 'Form in tonal motion', is probably the most concise. It also takes the most objective stance, regarding music as something distinct in itself – something 'over there'. His contemporary, the poet Heine was, however, less certain:

> Now, what is music? This question occupied me for hours before I fell asleep last night. Music is a strange thing. I would almost say it is a miracle. For it stands halfway between thought and phenomenon, between spirit and matter; a sort of nebulous mediator, like and unlike the thing it mediates – spirit that requires manifestation in time, and matter that can do without space. We do not know what music is. (tr. Nordoff and Robbins 1977)

A more modern definition is suggested by Thomas Clifton, 'Music is the actualisation of the possibility of any sound whatever to present to some human being a meaning which he experiences with his body – that is to say, with his mind, his feelings, his senses, his will, and his metabolism' (1983). He condenses this more aphoristically to 'music is what I am when I experience it'. This last statement by Clifton is nearer to the view of music which this book takes and, I hope, shows as having some validity.

One of the last things that Paul Nordoff said to a colleague visiting him when he was dying in hospital was 'You know, the greatest mystery of all is that we're made of music.' He had also often begun talking about music therapy to people by remarking that we ourselves are fundamentally rhythmic and tonal beings – music begins both with and *within* us. Thus our relationship to music is, in an important sense, of like to like and, as such, quite distinct from our relationship to spoken language.[1] We make and experience music because we have bodies which have pulses and tone, tensions and resolutions, phrasing of actions, bursts of intensity, repetitions and developments. Music gives us, in short, access to a whole world of experience: bodily, emotionally, intellectually and socially.

Music therapists confirm this basic view of music in every hour of their clinical practice, and all the case studies in this book emphasise how music is powerful (sometimes in the most extreme circumstances) because it 'gets inside us', because we 'become music' when we play and listen to it.

David Aldridge suggests that we should begin to think of ourselves as 'symphonic' beings rather than the mechanical ones that reductionist scientific medicine would often have us be (Aldridge 1989a, 1989b). We are, in more than just a metaphorical sense, continually 'composing' and 'improvising' ourselves as free agents in the world, with the psycho-physical self organising itself perhaps less like a machine and more like music. In his investigations into the correlations between music and our physiological and psychological functioning David Aldridge suggests that we have a basic *identity* with music. This is much more than saying someone is musical or not musical, that they can play or not. It suggests instead that music has, at a fundamental level, similarities of form and process with our psycho-physical functioning.

---

1 Though verbal language may be one of the most important defining features of us as human beings, music is possibly more essentially related to us as a whole organism. Indeed many of the case studies in this book illustrate that music can find access to people where words have failed.

In this way of understanding we do not merely hear and play, but have the prototypes of rhythm, melody, harmony and form in our physiological and psychological processes. An immediate objection to this idea might be that machines too have both frequency and repetition – the computer I write this on, for example, has an annoyingly loud fan with both of these features. Nevertheless, there is a qualitative difference that most of us intuit between mechanical noises and living things which can have 'pulse' and 'tone'. We can think of a heart beat or the tone of a voice (or, interestingly, the 'tone' of muscles – their degree of tension, reminding us of the strings of an instrument). It is then possible to see a hierarchy in complexity of these two elements, pulse and tone – from the purely biological to the artistic. At each level some further organisation[2] takes place.

Even at the basic biological level the flexible pulse of the heart is different from the rigid repetitive noise of a machine; the tone of the voice more than its invariant hum. Rhythm, however, is not just pulse but an organisation of events against a pulse. Rhythms begin to have some kind of identity which can be recognised and repeated in a short or longer period of time. Many of the body's systems also have an organisation which can be seen as essentially rhythmic: from the simple rhythms of short period – respiration, heart rate, peristalsis of the gut – to the longer periodic regulation of the autonomic and metabolic processes. As the anthropologist Lévi-Strauss expressed it somewhat more memorably, 'any piece of counterpoint includes a silent part for the rhythmic movement of heart and lungs' (Lévi-Strauss 1970).

In a similar way, tone can be organised as melody, a pattern of successive frequencies in time which are recognisable and repeatable. The body also has this need for the regulation of rising and falling frequencies. What could be called the 'melodic' aspects of functioning in the body organise those physiological events which have a more complex pattern of activity in time. Examples of this would be the fluctuations of temperature and hormonal release as well as the complex patterns of metabolic, cardiac and respiratory activity.

As in music, the 'rhythmic' and 'melodic' aspects of the self both serve to organise one element (such as respiration or temperature), whilst also allowing the synchronisation of one part with another. Within the body our different physiological rhythms are 'musically' entrained. Most of us have experienced a temporary failure of coordination when we have drunk too

---

2 'Organisation' is related to the concept of the 'organic', denoting something living as well as suggesting an increase of complexity and meaning.

much. But many illnesses involve a much more serious breakdown in the self-synchrony of the body. Music has been found by many people throughout the ages to be of help in these situations, when it seems to be able to bring about some synchronisation and order into both physical and mental life.

Oliver Sacks gives a powerful example of music as such a practical resource from his own personal experience. In his book *A Leg to Stand On* he describes how he damaged his leg in an accident in Norway. Coming down off the mountain in great pain his saving help was his ability to imagine music, 'There came to my aid now melody, rhythm and music (what Kant called the "quickening art"). Before crossing the stream I had "muscled" myself along. Now, so to speak, I was *musicked* along. I did not contrive this, it happened to me' (Sacks 1986). As the result of nerve damage he lost the natural 'feel' of movement in the leg, and the ability for spontaneous action. Unexpectedly, it was while a passage from Mendelssohn's Violin Concerto was running in his head that the leg was 'moved', in a different way from all his previous attempts to will it to move. Sacks describes that 'all of me, body and soul, became music in that moment'.

THE MUSIC BETWEEN US

There is not just a music within, but also one between us. In recent years the study of 'body language' has brought to our attention just how much of communication is non-verbal. Moreover, most of these non-verbal aspects of rapport with other people are grounded upon the rhythmic synchronisation or entrainment of our movements, speech and gestures – whether we are talking, making music or making love.

Awkwardness and dysynchrony, conversely, indicate a lack of effective communication. A famous study by Condon and Ogston consisted of the microanalysis of filmed conversations between mentally ill and 'normal' adults.[3] They investigated the characteristics of what they called 'interactional synchrony', the physical and expressive organisation of a communication, and suggested that even when two people are communicating in the alternating form of a verbal dialogue there is also a rhythmic 'dance' of rapport between them: 'The body of the speaker dances in time with his speech. Further, the body of the listener dances in rhythm with that of the speaker' (Condon and Ogston 1966).

---

3 This is described in greater detail in Chapter 15.

Speech and gesture have important rhythmic, dynamic and melodic aspects. As a melody gives shape and direction to tones, so our communicative gestures and words have intonation and phrasing. Again, both speaker and listener take part in this continual ebb and flow of shaped expression.[4] It was clear, however, that because mental illness seemed to interfere with self-synchrony and in the ability to use the 'musical' features of expression it also prevented effective communication between people. In short, that disturbance in self-synchrony interfered with 'interactional synchrony'. As David Aldridge writes:

> When the breakdown of this synchronous behaviour occurs then pathology is evident. The restriction of musical aspects of communication – pitch, stress, articulation, timbre and fluency – appear to be indicative of psychopathology. An improvement in these qualities appears to be evident in a return to health and the maintainance of a coherent identity. (Aldridge 1989b)

Unlike Condon and Ogston's study involving spoken conversations, a central characteristic of music-making is that two or more people can play at the same time. Indeed the complex synchronicity of music is one of its unique qualities. When people play music together there is at the same time a coordination of the music (its rhythms, melodies, harmonies) and of the bodies and minds of the players. There is the possibility of acting, thinking and feeling as one. As Leonard Bernstein said about conducting 'It's a love affair in which you and a body are pulsing together, lifting and sinking together.'

In a research project, music therapist Lutz Neugebauer collaborated with a physiologist to investigate what could be measured physiologically when two people improvise music together (Neugebauer 1992). The subjects were 'wired-up' to a heart monitor and the improvisation tape recorded. After the session the physiologist and music therapist separately analysed each of the datas from the point of view of their own professional criteria. In the case of the music therapist he listened for points of shared musical significance between the players – correspondences in rhythm, melody or phrasing. These points were then compared to the selection of interesting traces the physiologist had selected. It was clear that at the points of shared *musical* significance there was also a greater isomorphism between their physical

---

4 Mercedes Pavlicevic calls this overall process 'Dynamic Form'. More of this in Chapter 15.

processes. The depth of synchrony in musical communication is obviously deeper than we may imagine.

EMOTION AND MEANING IN MUSIC

An experiment which has a seemingly similar form was made with the conductor Herbert von Karajan, whose pulse rate was recorded both when conducting and whilst landing his private jet (Harrer and Harrer 1977). The first surprise in the results was that he showed more arousal conducting than landing the jet. But it is in the second finding that a warning lies against taking too mechanical a view about the relationship between music and physiology. It was found that, when conducting, it was not when Karajan's outer movement was most vigorous, but when he felt the most emotional response in a passage that his pulse showed the greatest increase.

This finding does not, I think, contradict our intuitions about music; that, in e.e. cummings' phrase 'feeling is first'. Consequently, the emphasis in this chapter on the physiological parallels with music is not to ignore the emotional aspects, but rather as a balance to the more commonly held belief that music is simply a language of the emotions. (I will go no further with this topic now, as there is a whole later chapter, 'Expressing', devoted to it.) Suffice to say here that the obvious correspondences between our emotional state and physiological arousal (when often conflicting emotions such as anger and excitement share the same form) are mirrored in the way music works. Our emotions share with music the qualities of speed, force, attack, intensity and so on. In this way bursting anger is mirrored in a burst of sound; depressed sluggishness in a slow aimless melody.

A second cautionary point about the ideas in this chapter is that in a sense it is a cheat to talk about rhythm and melody except as the components of organised music. One of the confusions that seeps into music therapy is that 'sound' is often mistakenly taken to be synonymous with 'music',[5] rather than the active ingredient which is given form and meaning as music. Nevertheless it is equally clear that it is not mere metaphor when we talk of the 'rhythm' of the heart or walking, or the 'melody' of a voice. To go back to Thomas Clifton's definition of music ('music is what I am when I experience it') what is important is perhaps not to look for an artificial dividing line between what is 'really' music and what is not, but to understand the relationship *between* 'sound' and 'music' and between music,

5 I use quotation marks with both of these words to indicate the difficulty in making any cut-and-dried definition.

the body and the mind. This is vital when we are investigating the phenomenon of music within music therapy, rather than in a more conventional musicological sense, when it is indeed easier to take a more objective view of musical phenomena.

The central fact of Creative Music Therapy is of two people sharing intention and meaning in music by improvising together. The physiological resonances operate within this, but the music and the communication *in* the music come from two minds finding meaning together. This happens through the musical components proper: of pulse and tone organised as rhythm and melody within a still higher organisation of phrasing, harmony and form.

By 'musical meaning' I do not suggest that the music represents anything else that can be put into words, images or even feelings. I mean that it is *meaningful*, that it makes sense in itself – that it connects together two minds, two bodies in the same experience. To take a somewhat unusual example from my own experience, I was on the London Underground one morning when the train stopped in a tunnel. Three people were strung out the length of the carriage, each immersed in their own world. After a time there was the sound of the train brakes, a shooshing noise. But it immediately became clear that it was an organised shooshing noise – the driver was 'playing' on the brakes the cliché rhythm below. The people in the carriage looked up

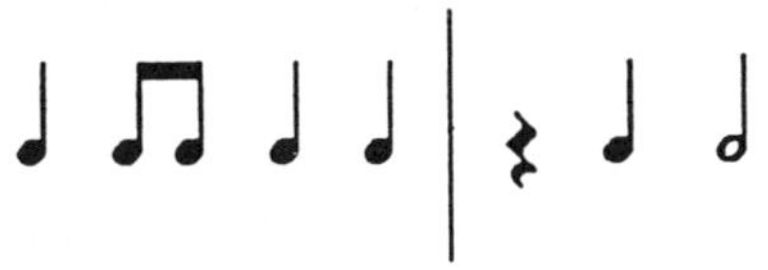

and smiled at each other in recognition of the joke. The 'music' was the pattern which connected the intention of the driver's mind with ours through the elements of rhythm and tone. A sophisticated piece of music it was not, and you could argue that this was just a signal, not music – that it gave an already conventional message. It was perhaps halfway between the purely signal function of a telephone bell and the creative complexity we expect of music.

Music involves an irreducible alchemy between mind and body, self and other. It can give us both a sense of transcending ourselves whilst simultaneously grounding us in our bodies and emotional life. We have, in the words of the French philosopher Merleau-Ponty, a 'complicity' with music, and it is the music therapist's job and skill to help anyone to the point where they can 'become music'; where music can act within and between them.

CHAPTER 2

Therapy in Art

> What strikes me is the fact that in our society, art has become something which is related only to objects and not to individuals, or to life. That art is something which is specialised or done by experts who are artists. But couldn't everyone's life become a work of art? Why should the lamp or the house be an art object, but not our life? (Michel Foucault)

The title of this chapter echoes that of Nordoff and Robbins' first book *Therapy in Music for Handicapped Children*. By choosing this they were emphasising how, in this approach, the therapy is part of the music rather than the music part of the therapy. What may seem a subtle distinction has become nevertheless a perennial issue in the arts therapies in general: the relationship between the art form and theories of therapy. The present chapter attempts to show how an art form can work within a specifically therapeutic context without, however, being automatically taken as just an artistic adjunct to verbal psychotherapy.

In her book *On Art and Therapy* Martina Thomson (1989) sounds the caution to art therapists that they should not lose sight of the fact that every one of the arts existed in its own right way before anyone developed the concept of art having a therapeutic value. And, in turn, art as therapy was working for people in this way before the professional art or music therapist arrived and considered him or herself essential to the process.[1] This caution warns us to approach any account of an arts therapy starting from the art form itself – its unique qualities and gifts – and only then look at how it is

---

1 None of the arts therapies has more than fifty years of tradition as organised professional disciplines.

possible to understand these within a specifically therapeutic context. This is not to deny the skill of the therapist but to make sure that we begin looking down the right end of the telescope when seeing how a 'therapy in music' (or any art) can be possible.

ART AS COMPENSATION

'There is no such thing as pessimistic art. Art affirms!' wrote Nietzsche. This feeling was echoed by a music therapy colleague I interviewed to collect a case study for this book. I asked him how he thought of his work with terminally ill clients. His answer was that, whilst the inevitable process of their illness and dying was essentially a downward spiral, the music therapy process always remained an upward one – it made contact, created meaning, affirmed life. Indeed, he and other music therapists have found that the intensity of a person's music-making often seems to increase as their physical energy decreases.

There is an old gypsy saying that music gives us what the rest of life denies us. This is movingly illustrated by Brian Keenan in his account of being kept hostage in Beirut for four and a half years. He writes how, after he had become almost numb and disconnected from his body, his memory produced almost as a hallucination, a symphony of all the music he had known for him to dance to:

> A tiny cell, a dozen candle stubs and a madman dancing naked. I was laughing. The laughter was part of the music around me. Not the laughter of hysteria, but the laugh of self-possession, the laugh that comes with the moment of victory. Every part of me, every limb, every muscle energized in this dance. (Keenan 1992)

In their extremity both this and the case of music therapy with terminally ill clients show a vital face of all the arts: that they both enhance what we have as potential within ourselves as well as compensating for what we lack. This is true in the general sense that they create order and meaning in the face of disorder and meaninglessness. But each of the art forms also has its own unique qualities which compensate for aspects of both our personal experience and of our culture. The order of music works against the disorder of noise; the grace of dance against stiffness and passivity; the liberation of images and metaphors against the dominance of concepts and measurements. Moreover, these qualities come not as some panacea applied to us, but as raw materials for our own creativity.

Despite this, contemporary culture puts the arts at arms length from most people's lives, a matter for the professional, the gifted, the creative. Art becomes consumed rather than experienced. But what of our own involvement, of making art ourselves, or more radically, of making ourselves art, as Foucault provocatively states in the epigraph to this chapter?

ART AS EXPERIENCE AND MOTIVATION

One of the few areas in our adult culture where art is not solely the province of the experts or the skilled amateur is within the arts therapies. Here there are approaches based on most of the art forms: art therapy, music therapy, dramatherapy, dance movement therapy. These are part of an answer to Foucault's question, for here a person can paint themselves, dance themselves, play themselves...free from many of the contraints that often inhibit our need to be creative.

Each of the arts therapies works essentially in the way its art form works. That is, music therapy is effective because of the unique qualities of music, dance therapy because of those of dance and so on. The skill of the therapist is to make that art, and the qualities of that art, accessible to the people they work with: whatever the physical or psychological obstacles. The range of case studies in this book show the imagination, resourcefulness and determination this often requires from the therapist. When the language of an art form is accessible then a person has the chance to be creative within it and for it to be the basis for a creative relationship between the therapist and client. The task of the therapist is to encourage, support and challenge this creative process.

Many arts therapies have also, however, taken on an additional dimension, where the need is felt to justify the work as 'therapy' not by virtue of the unique qualities each art is able to give a person, but by their inclusion into an established therapeutic theory and procedure. Thus many of the arts therapies are based on a psychodynamic[2] approach, involving both an explicit theory of human (psychological) disorder, and of the method of therapy. With this the creative experience within the art form (the music, dance or painting) is often taken as a starting point for verbal processing; the 'therapy' in the art is seen in terms of how this can yield material for analytic reflection. The danger here is that a person's experience of making music or painting becomes part of an explanation, rather than being allowed

2 'Psychodynamic' is used as a more generalised term for 'psychoanalytic'. Within the arts therapies it means any approach based on a psychotherapeutic model. This theme is expanded in the section 'How does Creative Music Therapy relate to psychotherapy?' in Chapter 4.

to represent itself in terms of its own unique qualities. I hope one of the messages of this book is that the arts as therapy can be allowed to work as the arts work for us in any context (be this private, public, educational or therapeutic): not to add to the store of our explicit knowledge but to extend the range and quality of our experience.

What all the art therapies *do* share in common, however, is the aim to involve people in creative action. Oliver Sacks (1990) remarks that one of the suggested derivations of the word 'inert' is from 'in-art', still visible in the modern word 'inarticulate'. Not to be acting is also not to be creating and developing in the world. What is interfering with a person's ability to articulate themselves can be as extreme as a handicap or a chronic illness, or as simple (but equally as paralysing) as a lack of confidence, or an inability to believe they *can* communicate spontaneously and creatively in music, art or dance.

What links together art and therapy are these shared beliefs in creativity and potential, in what *can be*, regardless of perceived limitations. But, as Oliver Sacks comments, the real function of art as therapy is not to instruct but to inspire. In his books he often talks about how powerful an experience it is for his patients with a neurological disorder (especially those living with Parkinson's disease) to be involved in music or dance. Music particularly seems to penetrate the passivity of the illness – it makes the person want to act. This quality of music which quickens the will led Sacks to comment that 'music has been the profoundest non-chemical medication for our patients' (Sacks 1991). He also talks of the art therapies as 'existence therapies' because they work directly on the will and on the existential areas of our experience where we find meaning and beauty. They work with what is integral to a person, not just their handicap or illness, 'One cannot have a Parkinsonian *person*: the "I" can never be 'Parkinsonianised'… Only by an existential approach can one liberate the "I" – the never-extinguished but dormant free-will or autonomy, which has been lying passive, enslaved by the "It"' (Sacks 1991). A danger in characterising art as a form of compensation is that it can seem too tame and open to a simplistic approach of almost prescribing the arts for people. As E.M. Forster remarked, the arts are not drugs. We also need to keep in mind the notion of the arts as a *challenge* to set ways of feeling, thinking or acting. Again there is no difference here between how the arts function within a specifically therapeutic context or within cultural life in general. As the literary critic George Steiner writes:

> The archaic torso in Rilke's famous poem says to us: 'Change your life'. So does any poem, novel, painting, musical composition worth meeting. The voice of intelligible form, of the needs of direct address

> from which such form springs, asks: 'What do you feel, what do you think of the possibilities of life, of the alternative shapes of being which are implicit in your experience of me, in our encounter?'. (Steiner 1989)

TWO INFLUENCES ON CREATIVE MUSIC THERAPY

Many of the above ideas are contained in two movements which have had some influence on the development of Creative Music Therapy – anthroposophy and the tradition of humanistic psychology.[3] In terms of the latter it was the influence of Abraham Maslow, who was part of the so-called 'third force' in psychology – a reaction against both Freudianism and behaviourism. Maslow became interested not just in people who were ill, but also those who did not become ill, who creatively fulfilled their potential. He investigated both the necessary conditions and the strategies people used to keep themselves healthy and happy. Being and staying creative he found to be one of the most important of these. Maslow looked at how spontaneous states such as joy, love and creativity have a motivating power which we all use, consciously or not, to enhance our psychological and physical well-being (Maslow 1976). He called these sometimes unexpected states 'peak experiences' and observed how they function to lift us out of our habitual modes and reactions and to help develop our intellectual and emotional life. Maslow referred to this developmental process as 'self-actualisation'. His ideas, and those of many who followed him, began to pave the way for a re-thinking of the dogmatic divide between science and art within the psychological and medical establishment.[4]

There is still, however, a real need for a view complementary to the 'medical model' for people who are ill or handicapped. Too often they still find themselves in a situation where scientific medicine treats them by continually measuring their deficits – the size of tumors, T-cell counts, movement capability, IQ and so on. The person being treated may feel that not only do they become a 'patient' (a term derived from 'passive') but also an object – that nobody sees them as a whole, with their problems *and* their potential. Within the arts therapies, however, exactly this happens: the person

---

3 With both of these approaches, however, it was the general message rather than any specific techniques which influenced the development of Creative Music Therapy at different stages.

4 Czikszentmihalyi has further developed this line of research. He characterises the quality of 'optimal experience' simply as 'flow' – a description any artist or arts therapist will recognise. (See Czikszentmihalyi 1988 and 1992.)

playing, dancing, painting themself can be seen and heard as a whole, something of *quality* rather than just quantity.

There are hopeful signs that at least some areas of the medical profession are interested in exploring what a qualitative and artistic perception of a patient can add to their clinical picture. It seems there is a gradual and necessary movement towards (more accurately perhaps a *return* to) what David Aldridge has called the *Art of Medicine* (Aldridge 1989b).

A philosophy which involves these ideas is anthroposophy, based on the ideas of Rudolf Steiner.[5] Nordoff and Robbins first met at a Sunfield Children's Home for handicapped children, run according to anthroposophic principles. The development of Creative Music Therapy was influenced by anthroposophic ideas regarding the use of the arts as therapy, and its emphasis on working with the whole person.[6] Anthroposophical medicine, for example, uses 'artistic therapies' as a complement to conventional and homeoepathic medication. The arts are used not as an entertainment but as part of a holistic approach to helping a person find a way of coping positively with their illness at all levels: body, mind and spirit (Evans and Rodger 1992). Arie Bos, an anthroposophical doctor working with people living with AIDS in Amsterdam, writes:

> Art is able to function as therapy, as a means to change. The essential aspect of recovery from a serious illness is change...the arts therapies are eminently suitable to enable the 'I' to become flexible enough to help bring about such a change, a new impulse which can act as a guiding light into the future. (Bos 1989)

Almost every case in this book is evidence of this point. The arts therapies in general, and Creative Music Therapy in particular, prepare the conditions where a person's potential can be motivated to unfold in its own unique way, and where growth can happen in its own time. The 'challenge' which George Steiner wrote about is inherent in the medium itself – some new quality that is required by playing, dancing, painting: 'What do you feel, what do you think of the alternative shapes of being which are implicit in me, in our

---

5 'Anthroposophical' is derived from the Greek 'anthropos' (human) and 'sophia' (wisdom). The anthroposophical movement defies neat categorisation but is basically a holistic metaphysical philosophy which nevertheless informs very practical areas such as medicine, education, agriculture and economics. In Britain it is known largely for its educational system, though on the continent the approach is also found in medical and therapeutic contexts.

6 There is also a substantially different form of music therapy called 'Anthroposophic Music Therapy' which works according to the anthroposophic world-view in a specific way.

encounter'. But there is also an ongoing challenge within the progressive therapeutic direction which the arts therapist always keeps in mind when working with a client. This is part of the answer to the question 'How can "just" playing music, dancing, painting be a *therapy*?' (especially when there is no verbal analysis), and how it differs from a single artistic experience.

THE 'SHAPE OF BEING'

In contrast to the set ranges and inflexibility of machines, one of our central characteristics as humans is the flexible range of our actions (from the purely physical to the creative). To call a person 'rigid' or 'inflexible' is seldom a compliment! When Nordoff and Robbins began working with handicapped children they analysed and compared the tapes of the sessions and one of the things they found common in the children was a shared limitation in the tempo and dynamic range in which they could beat a drum. Their handicap seemed to have narrowed their flexibility in playing music, and had therefore also narrowed their musical *experience*. Within the basic freedom of improvisation the therapists tried to extend the range and flexibility of the children's playing – encouraging through the music a wider range of tempo and other musical responses.

Since then music therapists working in this tradition have found a similar phenomenon occurring with other clients – whatever their age, ability or problem. Whilst it is difficult to say whether these 'tendencies of playing' are evidence of cause or effect, it is clear that the influence of the illness or the way of coping with the illness is often to narrow and limit in various ways the 'shape of being' as represented in a person's music. Rather than a deficit it is a loss of choice. Equally, many different factors get in the way of a flexible creative dialogue between people playing music together – the inability to listen; to hear anything outside of themselves; to tolerate the intimacy of playing with another person. These form the challenges posed by the dicatates of the music itself, and by the ongoing therapeutic relationship *in* the music. Within Creative Music Therapy and the arts therapies in general there is a subtle and irreducible interweaving of aesthetic and personal goals and of artistic and therapeutic developments.

Art does not force or coerce: it offers itself as a possibility. Therapy in art similarly offers a new form of experience; a new experience of form. This is art working as it works for all of us, but within the special and necessary conditions of a therapeutic context. For in every new experience of creativity, communication or beauty there can be a glimpse of the possibility of growth, potential and transcendence.

CHAPTER 3

Improvising

> In all its roles and appearances improvisation can be considered as the celebration of the moment. And in this the nature of improvisation exactly resembles the nature of music. Essentially, music is fleeting; its reality is in the moment of performance. (Derek Bailey)

During the last few years I have been commuting between two keyboards – a piano, on which to do music therapy, and a word-processor, on which to write about it. The end result of the not dissimular work of my fingers is of course two very different phenomena – words or tones. In his extraordinary study of learning to play jazz piano, *Ways of the Hand*, David Sudnow (1978) draws an interesting comparison between the two procedures. The beginner jazz pianist often starts by seeking patterned spatial 'pathways' on the piano keyboard in a similar way to how I now find my fingers 'finding' the pathways to type this sentence:

> It's almost as if you learned to keep on typing by using a rule like this: play every other key on the middle bank of characters; either go up, or down, up a bit then down a bit, up a bit then down a bit then up a bit more, and so on. You would get: adg dgj dgjl dgjljgd... (Sudnow 1978)

The result of this hand's 'pathway' is nonsense if we look for a semantic meaning in those 'words'. Interestingly, if Sudnow's example is taken one stage further and the typewritten letter patterns are converted into tones, the result (Figure 3.1) makes at least some musical sense.

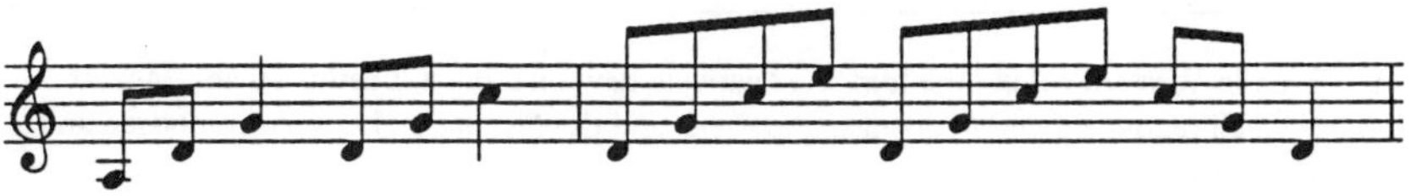

Figure 3.1

This rather odd example nevertheless illustrates something important about improvisation: that it rests on the specific and unique ways in which musical (as opposed to verbal) sense is made, and how the spontaneity of music can flow from the 'ways of the hand' and its patterns of order.

PLAYING IMMEDIATELY

Free improvisation is the main tool the music therapist has to involve someone immediately in a creative musical experience. By immediately, moreover, I mean not just in the sense of straight away (essential though this is). Starting with improvisation also means that playing music together need not necessarily be mediated by previous musical experience, skill on an instrument, or any particular level of mental or physical ability. Improvising allows music-making to begin at a level which is both suitable and possible.

Whilst a child or a mentally handicapped person will usually find it quite natural just to start improvising music, to a non-impaired adult it can sometimes seem a puzzling and intimidating idea. This is perhaps to do with the fact that improvisation is relatively unusual in our Western musical culture. Music as many people understand it is usually composed by a famous name and played by equally famous names, whose job it is to 'get it right'.[1] Even people familiar with folk, pop or jazz musics tend still to regard the music as something 'over there', to be played by someone else. It is a novel idea to them that you can improvise your own music on the spot.

At the other extreme, a client of mine called David (a blind man whose story appears later in the book) fell around laughing when I explained to him that music could be written down on a piece of paper and played again. Yet around 90 per cent of the world's musicians would basically agree with David. Further, if you asked them whose music they played the answer would probably be 'my own, of course!' A recent series of television programmes called *On the Edge*, based on Derek Bailey's (1992) book *Improvisation*, travelled around the musical world – from jazz, rock, and folk to the sophisticated ancient traditions of North Indian classical music, from flamenco to the music of a remote African village. The thread that linked these very diverse musical cultures was that improvisation was central to all of them. It is the Western classical tradition that is the odd man out – where

---

1 Even in Western culture the idea is a relatively new one. Bach, Beethoven and Mozart were all renowned and frequent improvisers, and the distinction between composed and improvised music less sharp.

everything is predetermined, where the player's task is to reproduce rather than to create.

Improvisation to Ravi Shankar, Keith Jarrett or Paco Peña is not just an occasional freedom, but a whole approach to the creation and performance of music. They would probably think of themselves creating their own personal testament in a performance, be it one firmly rooted in a tradition or an idiom. This is quite different from, for example, the way a concert pianist would think about a performance they were giving of a Beethoven concerto. Though probably hoping that they were giving a technically proficient and musically sensitive interpretation of the piece, they would certainly *not* think of how creative they were being with the notes! This aspect has already been predetermined and fixed in the score. In the Western classical tradition the roles of the creator and of the performer have been separated. I am not saying this is intrinsically bad, but it has nevertheless influenced our attitudes about what music 'should' be.[2]

Yet the very way in which improvisation differs from mainstream music-making in our culture makes it a vital tool for Creative Music Therapy. The title from the television series on improvisation was taken from a remark made by the jazz player Steve Lacey, 'There's a certain quality, which can only be obtained from improvisation, something you cannot possibly get from writing. It is something to do with the "edge". Always being on the brink of the unknown, and being prepared for the leap' (Bailey 1992). For the music therapy clients who come to us for the first time it is certainly a leap, but one that mostly ends with unexpected flight. My approach in the first session is usually the same. After a few initial formalities I will give the client a single drumstick as they stand in front of a side-drum and cymbal (at a reasonable distance from me on the piano). I then usually say something like 'away we go then – you just start playing any way you want, and I'll join in!' There is no preparation, no instruction – we simply begin straight away and, within seconds usually, we are improvising music together.

I would probably use this same procedure for a first session whether the client was an autistic child or an adult who was a professional violinist. People very occasionally remark that it seems childish, that it reminds them of school music. But the only significance of the drum and cymbal arrangement is that it is the easiest pair of contrasting sounding instruments to play. Someone,

2 There have, however, been some unexpected improvisers among amateur musicians. Einstein is reported to have claimed that it was both an emotional and an intellectual necessity for him to improvise daily. Nietzsche, in his final madness would improvise on the piano for himself when he could no longer talk.

whatever their skill or condition, can come in and immediately start making music and creating a musical dialogue with the therapist, without first having to master a complex instrument. Later, as the sessions progress, we move on to other instruments – xylophones, gongs, tuned and untuned percussion, piano duets, singing.

BEYOND 'RIGHT' AND 'WRONG'

The word 'improvisation' means 'not being able to see through'. The music is created in the performance and, by its nature, is unforeseen, undetermined and unpredictable; a daring to create from the conditions of the present moment, without knowing where the journey will lead. A member of the music therapy group written about later in this book said:

> Sometimes, when I was really flowing, the music seemed to play itself through me. These were the most exciting times for me. Perhaps you might say that my inner musician was allowed out fully to *play*. I could appreciate the thrill that jazz musicians must feel as they improvise. It is just satisfying in a way complete unto itself. I knew it was good for me by how well I felt afterwards.

To be fair, no improvisation is totally unpredictable. An improviser has in his or her head and fingers the style and repertoire of a musical tradition. But in improvisation there is always the space for the unexpected. Whilst the Western classical tradition furiously notates everything so that nothing is ever left to chance, improvisation allows for the sudden inspiration, when in the moment of performance the human creative imagination unexpectedly rises to chance.

My own favourite example of this is a ten-second stretch in the recording of one of the jazz pianist Keith Jarrett's solo piano improvisations. Jarrett has set up a repetitive ostinato pattern in his left hand, but then seems to miss the 'right' note (according to the pattern). However, he has such musical flexibility that he instantly uses the 'mistake' to create something new – starting the next repetition of the figure on the 'wrong' note and 'correcting' it upwards. This does not sound like a mechanical correction but an inspired detail which then changes the course of the music. This small example seems to me nothing less than a paradigm for what happens in improvisation.

Jarrett's 'wrong note' episode also shows another vital quality of improvisation: that it cannot be right or wrong, it is simply what happens. Another member of the music therapy group commented, 'I had to fight the belief that there is a "right" and a "wrong" way to do everything and this seemed an enormous opportunity to get it "wrong".'

When Nordoff and Robbins began music therapy it was this aspect that was unusual in their work with children with special needs. Previously people had, as a rule, taken in prepared music to play for or with the children, expecting them to fit into musical activities with an already fixed form. But this instantly creates a situation where right and wrong becomes an issue. If a piece is pre-set it is the person who must fit in, must play or sing a particular note at a particular moment. In most situations where music therapy is needed, however, such an approach is often counter-productive.[3]

Instead, Nordoff and Robbins began from the opposite angle, with free improvisation as their tool, inviting the child simply to play. Nothing could be right or wrong, but equally anything could happen. For the children they worked with, improvisation was often the only way to establish a channel of communication through the music. Improvised music can be tailored to meet the needs of the minute. Even if a client is unable or unwilling to play an instrument, I can improvise music to meet the timing of a rocking body or a pattern of breathing. There is always the possibility of some point of musical contact, however small and fleeting this may at first be.

I remember one client of mine, an autistic man, whose only response during the two years I saw him weekly was a tapping of his foot and a blinking of his eyelashes, to which I would entrain the music I improvised. I had to watch these movements out of the corner of my eye since he would instantly stop if he thought I had noticed. Though an outsider might well see no communication between us I always had the strong sense that there was a very real contact between him and myself in the music. I persevered because I knew that this was probably the only intimate contact R. could bear in his shadowy world. Without improvisation it would have been impossible.

Though this was perhaps an extreme example, music therapists often work with clients who at first seem very isolated and uncommunicative. Nevertheless, a point of contact can nearly always be found through improvisation, leading to an ongoing musical dialogue which can be intimate, creative and developing.

---

3 This is not to say that there is a taboo against pre-composed material in Creative Music Therapy. Nordoff and Robbins used their own and others' pieces, especially in group work. Equally many therapists incorporate songs into sessions when appropriate. The important point is that even then the 'philosophy' is an improvisational one – the emphasis being not necessarily on the song for its own sake, but for its use in music-making as a whole.

THE GIFTS AND DEMANDS OF IMPROVISATION

Though improvisation is a necessity for working with people like R. and some of the children with whom Nordoff and Robbins worked, it is also important for those clients who are in less extreme situations or who are quite capable of fitting into a pre-set musical structure. It is precisely the qualities of immediacy and unpredictability which are valuable therapeutically even to the trained musician coming to music therapy. Or perhaps I should say *especially* to the trained musician, since he or she has often lost some of the creative, personal connection to music due to the demands of professional playing.

Improvisation by-passes people's habit of thinking things out, of worrying whether a thing is right or wrong, of determining what will or should happen. The experience that improvising music with another person gives us is much the same for the handicapped child, the musically untrained adult and the professional musician: being involved immediately in the process of music-making; communicating intimately with another person through creatively improvising musical meaning with them.

'Musical meaning' is not the same as a verbal meaning, however. Whether it is in a pre-composed piece or in the development of an improvisation, music contains and continually creates meaning within itself rather than beyond itself. The confusion comes when people try to compare the way music works with the way verbal language works. Words always point to something beyond themselves – their whole *raison d'être* is to *refer* to things. In contrast music, rather than 'having a meaning' becomes *meaningful* as one or more people build a structure of rhythms, melodies and harmonies within an overall form. We communicate with words to convey our meaning, whereas we improvise music to *find* something meaningful between us:

> What happens is that by improvising meaningfulness, by each contribution that's made towards this improvised meaningfulness, you make things more meaningful. It's a bootstrapping process; you bootstrap it up from nothingness, and create a contingent somethingness. And each time someone does something more in the way of improvising purpose it actually is a permanent contribution towards it. (Jonathan Miller, in Dinnage 1992)

Keith Jarrett wrote that 'music's about your blood flowing, and can you feel it, and if so can you now translate what that means?' (Carr 1992). Jarrett's biographer, Ian Carr, writes about his characteristic physical identification with his music – of 'true improvisation that is actual creation in the process of an instrument done with the musician's sense of his own flow of himself' (Carr 1992).

In music therapy it is this sense of flow of both the music and the self which is often an unusual and fulfilling experience for our clients. The close identification of the person and the music allow the therapist to hear the client 'in' the music in a very precise way. We can see ourselves, like music, as a form that is continually being improvised in the world, and consequently the improvisation is a manifestation not only of a purely musical logic and style, but also of the client's unique physical, mental and social condition at that time. Though the main function of Creative Music Therapy is not as a diagnostic method, this hearing of a client in the music can be a valuable guide to the needs and direction of the therapy.

The gifts of improvisation – immediacy, involvement, unpredictability – are balanced by the demands it makes: to listen, to be aware, to dare to create; to remain in the present. These are the very opposite of some of the tendencies of many of our clients, to a lesser or greater extent. They are often lost in the past or the future (as habit or anxiety); have lost the ability to listen to themselves or others and tend to have rigid and inflexible patterns of behaviour.

In contrast, improvisation in a music therapy context encourages and cultivates the qualities of awareness, listening and creativity. When music involves, and improvisation seizes the present, there can emerge the opportunity for a person to experience themself differently from their habitual state.

Colin Lee's client, Francis, told him 'The only moment that I really feel that I'm living the time that I've got left is when I'm improvising [music with you]... It's the only time that I feel I am alive and communicating and living.'

CHAPTER 4

Nothing but Tones

> What is man, that this almost-nothing, this 'nothing but tones', could be one of his most significant experiences? (Victor Zuckerkandl)

At the end of this introductory section of the book it may be clear just how ambiguous the role of the music therapist is: how music therapy straddles ideas of art and ideas of therapy, and how the music therapist is called to reconcile a double role. Whilst this may not be conducive to providing cut-and-dried explanations of the music therapy process, the ambiguity does provide a rich new territory for investigation.

This far I have presented the basis of Creative Music Therapy as coming not from any pre-existing theory but from a process of observation of how music can work for people. Further, I believe that the process need not rely on extra-musical theories in order to explain itself. At the same time it is clear that there are nevertheless many aspects which Creative Music Therapy *does* share with other therapeutic and treatment systems (see Ruud 1980). It would indeed be impossible to have a music therapy which was not aligned, in however subtle a way, to a set of beliefs and values concerning people and music. Creative Music Therapy differs from many other approaches to music therapy in emphasising the purely musical underpinning of the work – before (if at all) this is placed in the context of any further model of health, illness or therapy. This last chapter of Part One attempts to distinguish between the aspects Creative Music Therapy shares in common with other types of music therapy, music-making and treatment approaches and those aspects which are significantly different.

THE THERAPEUTIC CONTEXT

Experience has taught therapists of a variety of persuasions a few basics of practice: that stability in the time and place of the sessions, and a dependability in the therapist are often necessary to establish the trust and ease of the client. Equally general will be the fact that the therapist will have both experience and an understanding of the process he works with, allowing him to support and perhaps guide the client through any possible changes and developments (technical and personal) which may come about through the therapeutic process. His actions need not be based on a rigid theory or be an obviously directive process. Indeed they may be based more on what to avoid, rather than being a pro-active strategy.

But none of these supporting aspects is the essence of the process, or even necessary at all. In Mathew's case (see Chapter 25), for example, continuity of the therapist was not his main need. He was equally happy with anyone who would work in a similar way with him. Mathew was there primarily for the music. Who happened to be providing the context for the music-making was undoubtedly secondary to him. Equally, many of the kind of experiences described in the case histories in this book also happen outside of the specialised context of music therapy – as the example of Oliver Sacks and others I quote later testify.

SOME QUESTIONS AND ANSWERS

The divergence between Creative Music Therapy and other therapeutic approaches and disciplines is not, however, so easily explained. This section is based around some of the most common questions we are asked – which, not surprisingly, encapsulate the main areas of confusion. The questions and answers which follow tackle issues concerning the relationship between Creative Music Therapy and ideas about therapy in general, and Creative Music Therapy and other music therapy approaches. The comments here are intended as introductory spurs to thought which are developed and substantiated in the essay chapters of Parts Two and Three.

How does Creative Music Therapy relate to psychotherapy?

Both the ideas of psychotherapy and the image of how it works are now so powerfully woven into our culture that music therapy is often assumed to be psychotherapy with a musical element. And indeed, several approaches to music therapy do work from a psychodynamic understanding of the therapeutic process. Similarly, other arts therapies have intentionally subsumed themselves within a general psychotherapy 'umbrella' (one art therapy training recently having changed its title to 'Art Psychotherapy'). Creative Music Therapy, however, is significantly different from a 'music psychotherapy'. It is not based upon either the principles or the procedures of psychodynamic theory and cannot be adequately explained by it.[1]

People come to both the psychotherapist and the music therapist for professional help: to the psychotherapist mainly because of psychological distress, to a music therapist also possibly because of physical problems resulting from a disability or chronic illness. Both therapists try to establish a secure, trusting relationship with the client, which can sometimes extend over years. Both want to encourage and support any changes that may happen to the client. But beyond these similarities in the overall aims of the therapy and in the context in which it takes place, there are important differences. In short it could be said that psychotherapy is a 'hermeneutical', and Creative Music Therapy a 'phenomenological' approach.[2] This in turn rests upon the essential difference between music and words. We need both of course, but they work in different ways both within our everyday life and within therapy. The musicologist Victor Zuckerkandl highlighted the difference, 'Words divide, tones unite. The unity of existence that the word constantly breaks up, dividing thing from thing, subject from object, is constantly restored in the tone' (Zuckerkandl 1976). Psychotherapy uses words to divide. It is rightly called a process of *analysis* which takes apart our experiences and personal construction of the world – our thoughts and feelings – in order to examine them. Its motto is the Socratic groundrule 'the unexamined life is not worth living', and its tool for this examination the word. Despite all the non-verbal and symbolic refinements, psychotherapy still retains its basic identity in Freud's original 'talking cure'.[3] Psychotherapy works through language, but it also works in the way that language works. The way the

---

1 Psychodynamic theory stems from the psychoanalytical tradition of Freud, Jung etc. Its theory of mental life as expressed in human behaviour is based around the 'dynamic' forces of instinctual drives and unconscious motives. In psychodynamic work the analyst makes (mostly verbal) interpretations of the expressions of patients, to help them to a greater understanding of the grounds of their behaviour, feelings and thoughts.
This is not to say, however, that the insights of individual analysts (such as Jung and Winnicott) into the therapeutic process, creativity etc. may not provide the music therapist with valuable ideas. The point is that it does *not* provide a complete explanatory model.

2 Hermeneutics is a 'reading' of something – it interprets, translates decodes. The psychoanalyst offers his 'reading' of the symbolism of a statement or dream. Likewise a hermeneutics of music tries to express verbally the 'meaning' of the music – what it represents. In contrast a phenomenology tries to understand a thing in its own terms – resisting interpretation. In Creative Music Therapy the focus of the work and any explanation is phenomenological – needing no verbal account but allowing the music to 'mean itself'.

3 'Nothing takes place in a psychoanalytic treatment but an interchange of words between the patient and the analyst' (Freud 1951).

client communicates his or her past experience is a verbal narrative, whilst the interpretations the therapist may make are, like the foreign language interpreter, a 'putting in other words' or a redescription.

In contrast music acts to unite, and Creative Music Therapy works in the same way as music works. The client needs no verbal competence for music therapy to be possible. If words take us apart, then music puts us together – physically, emotionally, mentally and socially. It acts to synthesise, not to analyse.

Creative Music Therapy developed because words were unavailable. Nordoff and Robbins' work was with handicapped and psychotic children who often had little or no language. Instead they found music to be the bridge of communication and meaning in establishing a long-term therapeutic relationship. In Creative Music Therapy there are no verbal instructions before the improvisations between the client and therapist, and there are no interpretations afterwards.

A child or a mentally handicapped adult will usually be quite happy to accept the musical experience for what it is. Many music therapists, however, also see clients who *are* verbal and who have an inner life of words, symbols and concepts, and who have preconceptions of what therapy 'should' be. How, then, do these clients react to a purely musical music therapy which does not involve verbal processing? Some are indeed disconcerted at first – they wonder how it can be effective if words and concepts are not being used to analyse the experience. Others are relieved to be free of words for a time. A member of a music therapy group I ran said 'I feel understood here when we're playing music together, in a way I never feel when I'm communicating with words.' Most clients seem to reach a stage when they allow themselves to experience what Creative Music Therapy *can* do and not worry about what they think it ought to be.

A central and distinguishing feature of musical experience is the sense of being involved, of being 'lost' in the present. Only words have past tenses; music must be in the here and now.[4] Psychotherapy's use of words to explore the past, to ask 'why?' questions of motive and significance is quite different from Creative Music Therapy's use of music to create a musical experience of the present. Its questions are rather 'what?' questions – What is happening now? What is the character and what are the qualities of the music we are able to create together here and now? For it is this quality of the musical

---

4 This statement perhaps needs qualifying. Music can certainly *evoke* the past: but the process of making music grounds us in the present.

dialogue which is central to the client's experience of the therapy *in* music. The heart of the therapy is contained within the music – an experience which is allowed to speak for itself.

Is Creative Music Therapy a behaviourist approach?

Behaviourism,[5] though a very different theory from psychodynamic psychotherapy, is nevertheless an equally misleading model when applied to creative therapies in general and to Creative Music Therapy in particular.

Largely in America there have been approaches to music therapy which conform to behaviourist theory. Music here is usually the reward (or 'reinforcement') for the completion of a particular desired piece of behaviour within a 'behaviour modification programme' for mentally handicapped children or adults. The music is usually played to the person from a tape – no creativity is involved. Representative of this would be an example quoted by Ruud (1980), from the American *Journal of Music Therapy* entitled 'Programmed Use of Music to Alter Uncooperative Problem Behaviour'. This kind of work was partly a response to pressure on some American music therapists to undertake 'outcome' trials in which the effectiveness of music therapy could be evaluated statistically. Statistics, however, cannot measure the quality of human contact, creativity or joy. Most behaviourist music therapy is both limited musically and limiting to its clients. It fails to make use of the riches of live music-making to reach the potential of music therapy.[6]

In comparison, however, to some styles of 'non-directive' music therapy, Creative Music Therapy seems to be quite interventionist in its approach, and it is suggested occasionally that it has subtle behaviourist tendencies. This is not meant as a compliment! Someone could, for example, be observing a session with a child who is responding very little. The therapist, however, is still playing music and seems almost to be demanding a response from the child (that he play the drum). In contrast to a behaviourist programme though, the therapist is not trying to condition a particular appropriate response from a predictable stimulus. Instead the *music* motivates the child's will to communicate and to respond not reflexly but creatively.

---

5 I use the term not to denote the academic psychological science but the therapeutic applications that developed out of this model, such as 'behaviour modification'.

6 'Behaviourists have neglected the study of inner personal meanings – purposes, goals, values, choice, perceptions of self, perceptions of others, the personal constructs with which we build our world, the responsibilities we accept or reject, the whole phenomenal world of the individual with its connective tissue of meaning' (Ruud 1980).

Any musical response that forms the basis of musical dialogue is evidence of a freely willed, intentional force directed from the inner world to the outer. It is a demonstration of the very inner, unconditional and dynamic forces that behaviourism would like to exclude from its picture of human functioning.

Behaviourism, in whatever guise, works towards the goal of the 'normalisation' of a person. But this makes a mockery of both the creative process and of the inner potential of a person to develop in a way perhaps unforeseen and unpredicted. Nordoff and Robbins were explicit about this in their work, 'A therapy that has as a goal the freeing and development of the individual within universal human principles is more effective than one which merely aims to normalise' (Nordoff and Robbins 1971). In Creative Music Therapy there is no aim to 'normalise', to get a desired pattern of musical behaviour. Instead there is a respect for that which is human and valuable in every person in all his or her individuality.

How does Creative Music Therapy relate to 'New Age' ideas about music?

There are now a profusion of workshops, books and tapes on a wide variety of techniques such as 'toning', chanting (Christian to Mongolian) and 'healing through sound' methods. Many people ask what the connection is between this exotic variety of approaches and the work of most professionally trained music therapists.

Many 'sound healing' techniques explain themselves with reference to a larger set of beliefs, be these spiritual or medical, Eastern or Western. From these derive theories about the influence of sound on the physiology of the body and on mental states. My intention here is not to evaluate these approaches but to make a comparison with Creative Music Therapy.

One of the confusions comes through considering sound and music as synonymous. Though we must not fall into the trap of making a definition of music too exclusive, nevertheless not all sound is music, and not all making of sound is music-making. Sound can be anything from a beautiful Greek bell to the sound of a juggernaut. The effect of pure sound can undoubtedly be beneficial – from the surgeon's use of 'Ultrasound' to the spiritual resonance of chanting. But music is more than sound, and it is what communicative significance is made out of sound as *music* that is the real concern of music therapy.

Music is sound organised by a human mind with the intention of 'meaning' something to another human mind, and is profoundly communicative in its potential for variety, creativity and complexity. In music therapy, where the client and therapist are improvising music together, music invites a response and can adapt to that response. 'Sound therapies' by contrast are usually 'applied' to a person who is passive. They may provoke a reaction, but mostly they invite no response.

Another tendency of the 'New Age' use of music which is alien to the approach of Creative Music Therapy is that of 'prescribing' music in the same way as any other medical remedy. For example, in a recent book Bradford Weeks, an American doctor writes 'perhaps the MD of the future will refer patients with infections, depressions or cancer to a music therapist for specific therapeutic tonal experience' (Campbell 1991).

This is simply too reductionist, of both music and therapy. As E.M. Forster wrote, 'the arts are not drugs, they are not guaranteed to act when taken. Something as mysterious and capricious as the creative impulse has to be released before they can act' (Sacks 1991).

The creative musical relationship in the music is part of a whole matrix of communication, meaning, thought and feeling shared with another person. More importantly, music therapy has no aim to cure. What it can do, and often achieves perhaps more than any other intervention, is to *alleviate*[7] a person as a whole – body, mind and spirit. Therapists in Creative Music Therapy work with that part of a person which is still well and creative, and can rise above the limitations of the illness or handicap.

Is Creative Music Therapy a special form of music teaching? Is it more than just entertainment?

Another one of the convenient boxes the music therapist is put into is that of 'special education'. It is often assumed that she is teaching music to a child or an adult with learning difficulties. But music therapists also take clients who are professionally trained musicians. They consult us because of a problem, but not one of technical proficiency. Indeed their musical skills may well be superior to those of the therapist.

People often ask how much musical skill you need to have music therapy as a client. My answer is 'the amount of skill you have now'. The fact that the autistic child has a very different level of skill from the trained musician makes little difference to the essential process of Creative Music Therapy. They both have a similar experience.

What the music therapist is *not* doing is fostering musical skill as a primary aim (as a music teacher does). If, as a result of music therapy sessions, clients

---

7 From the Latin 'to make lighter'. Quite often people report their experience of improvising as feeling lighter or 'flying'.

happen to improve their ability to play drums, for example, then that is fine, but it is not the aim of the therapy.

Teachers aim to add something to their pupils (a new level of skill or knowledge) whilst the therapist attempts to provide the right conditions for the client to experience themselves in a different way – where the physical, emotional or social conditions which limit their life are moderated. One of the meanings of the word 'therapist' is someone who accompanies, who helps a person make their own journey of exploration and experience.

Most music therapists have suffered at some point from being put down as a glorified entertainer, just as most psychotherapists will have been asked whether they are really better than finding a friend to talk to when you have a problem. Which is not to say that entertainment is *not* part of music therapy – playing music with another person is indeed often entertaining and joyous. But whatever the character of the experience, it happens, as does the verbal dialogue of psychotherapy, within a sustained, secure and dependable relationship. Therapy is based on the premise of growth and development allowed to unfold naturally in its own time. Music is a powerful phenomenon as entertainment pure and simple. It is also a powerful agent within the specific context of therapy.

At the end of this part of the book entitled 'What is Creative Music Therapy?' I have resisted making a definition until the eleventh hour, in order to build up the picture gradually rather than present it ready-framed in the first sentence. It is not, however, difficult to define this approach in relatively simple terms. The aim of Creative Music Therapy is to benefit people by giving them access to a creative music relationship within a sustained and dependable therapeutic context. I attempt to outline how this happens in practice in Part Two.

Part Two

What Happens in Creative Music Therapy?

Introduction

Having outlined aspects of the background of Creative Music Therapy and to some extent what Creative Music Therapy is *not*, the remainder of this book now turns to what it is: which needs not just ideas and principles but the musical stories of people.

The question I kept asking myself and the colleagues I interviewed for the case histories was, how does music act *within* this person, and how does it act *between* people in a music therapy context? Sometimes this is an easy question to answer. To a person with learning difficulties isolated by a lack of verbal ability, music and music therapy gives access to an intimate, creative dialogue with another person. To a person 'frozen' by a neurological illness music gives 'quickness', a feel of life and movement. To someone living with a mental health problem it can give a meaningful sense of contact and purpose through creating something with another person.

These aspects come out in the case histories themselves, but they are also supplemented in Part Two by short essays on some of these ideas: on 'meeting' (the contact established in the music), creating, listening; and on the unique qualities of music which help to 'quicken' and 'recall' people whom illness and handicap have put on the edge of human experience. This work, however, has equally important implications for the people who are by no means in an extreme condition, but who find in music therapy a new dimension of communication, expression and creativity within themselves.

A certain artificiality comes in separating out the various aspects of the whole process of music therapy. But in another way the separation makes sense, since each aspect is part of a progressive order, with each dependent on the previous stage having been established. Thus improvisation makes musical contact possible; which allows an improvised dialogue to develop; which allows a creative process of developing musical structure, and so on.

But, equally, both the qualities of the music, and the 'processes' of Creative Music Therapy mostly happen together. Like a piece of music itself the music therapy process is a counterpoint of the different themes of the nature of music and musical interaction.

Part Two attempts to show both the progression and the simultaneity in the music therapy process: what can be taken out of the work as principle and ideas and what can only be told through the musical stories of people.

CHAPTER 5

Emanuella

> The road is there, but we do not necessarily go along it, but may walk round and round the same point, unable to escape the circle of our own habits. (Maurice Nicoll)

For the two-and-a-half years that I saw Em our first quarter of an hour from 4.30 every Friday afternoon was a largely unvarying script. As I entered the sitting room she took a few minutes to recognise me (though I was told she had been anticipating my arrival for hours), and our script began:

'Hi Em!'

(*shouts*) 'GET OWT! GO AVAY!'

'That's not a very nice welcome…'

'I know. I don't want eet. I will call a policeman…'

'Ah, but I thought you had a good time playing last week…'

'I hate Gary, I hate museek, I hate eet…'

'Oh dear, shall we just do a bit?'

'No. You are the rubbish! I won't play…'

'I tell you what, I'll get the instruments ready and I'll just play you some music. OK?'

'OK.'

Emanuella had a thick central European accent which she used to full emotional effect in the prelude to each of our sessions. I was taken aback by the force of her rejection of me at first, but after a while, when I had seen the whole pattern, I accepted it as part of the inevitable drama.

Em refused to go out so I had to visit her at home, where she lived in a friendly house with four other women with learning difficulties. I was surprised to learn that she was fifty-five, old even these days for a person living with Down's Syndrome. Yet Em looked a lot younger than her years, with her soft round face above an equally short and round body. She and her mother had come to England during the war as refugees, and it was thought there were some traumatic incidents in her early life. After her mother's death she had joined the community home where she was much loved despite the frustration she often caused.

Our opening script was usually played in the sitting room as I prepared the instruments. Repetitive as it was, this was one of the easy days. A bad day was when she fled to her bedroom at the sound of me at the doorbell. There was a long period where Em voiced her resistance to me and music therapy by taking all her clothes off and preparing for bed at 3pm. I then had to persuade her to come back into the other room (where the piano and instruments were) against the full force of her obsessional habits. I stopped taking all this personally when I found out that Em meted out the same treatment to almost everyone, and that evidently in comparison to the rabbi I was let off comparatively lightly! I also learnt that the severity of the refusal was no index of whether she did want something or not. She simply rejected everything at first. It was part of an overall pattern of Em's behaviour that had contracted her life into a tight ball of ritual habits and fearful rejections of anything new or unknown. Em's day itself had gradually contracted as she refused to get up until midday and then, after all the ritual preparations had been completed, it was only a matter of hours before she started to reverse this process in order to go to bed again. Many an agonised Friday afternoon I watched the routine for slowly edging into the room where we did the music: folding day clothes, preparing night clothes, edging up the bed (left to right) by the inch, stroking the doorknob eleven times. All this was accompanied by an equally ritual argument with Dora, Em's room-mate.

Despite the resistance it was usually the exception when Em did not, of her own choice, finally make it into the other room when the ritual cycle was complete. In comparison to most of the other case studies in this book I have gone into considerable detail in describing how Em was in the world *outside* music. This is to emphasise the contrast with how she was *'inside'* music and a musical relationship. It also represents the balance of time within the session: of the hour I spent weekly with Em half an hour was spent preparing for the music, and half successfully playing. You may well be thinking at this stage that my continuing for this time with an activity Em seemingly didn't want was for both of us a waste of time and emotional energy. But I can honestly say that the second half hour always justified the first.

The sitting room was long and narrow with the piano at one end, besides which I set up a chair and a drum. Em always retreated to the very opposite end of the room and sat on the end of the sofa. My gentle hello-song was usually punctuated by less than positive interjections from Em, which on a bad day increased to loud shouts which reverberated around the rest of the house [☉1]. A later variant went:

'Hello, hello Emanuella...'

'SHUTUP! No–Gary–No, I won't play! I don't deserve eet!'

This last expression I took to be a gesture of modesty to which I countered 'Of course you do, Em!' It was only later that I discovered, from one of the care assistants, that I had misunderstood. What she meant was that she did not deserve such (bad) treatment! However, as I persevered with the song, the interjections became fewer and I could see out of the corner of my eye that Em's face was softening. The music was melting the resistance.

After the hello-song I generally improvised on the piano in a faster tempo. Em was one of the clients I have worked with who was inspired by particular characters of music. Perhaps predictably, it was my attempt at a typical Jewish dance-music style which caught not just her attention but also her body. She did occasionally burst out singing fragments of what I took to be Yiddish songs, but I never followed this up in any specific way. With Em it seemed so important that whatever music we made it had to be totally in the present, not a reconstruction of the past, as most of her everyday life was. However, this style obviously had emotional resonances for her and was another help to get around the ever-present resistance.

Sometimes the shouting (NO!–NO!–NO!) would still be going on, but timed with the music in metrical blows on the coffee-table with a rolled-up copy of the *Jewish Chronicle.* On a gentler day Em would start clapping her hands or I would see her foot tapping to the music, then the *Jewish Chronicle* surreptitiously tapping on the sofa. I followed her starts and stops: she would look out of the corner of her eye to see if I knew that she knew... [☉2]

Despite playing, Em still kept a resolute five-yard distance from me and the drum. In frustration I sometimes offered a verbal invitation: 'How about playing the drum for a bit, Em?', to which my answer was usually, 'No–Gary–No...I won't play the drum today. Go home!' Instead I placed the drumstick temptingly on the drum and continued playing – incorporating any musical responses Em made into the improvisation, but being careful not to pose too direct a challenge. Em would always weaken and come over, usually with a little dance, arms held up each side to her head, body swaying. The arrival at the drum I tried to treat as a surprise rather than a victory. As she took the drumstick she would often still be muttering 'I won't play, not today, no I won't.'

But she did, and from the confident first burst of drum we generally played for twenty to thirty minutes non-stop. Em's playing was actually quite limited. She had a tendency to get stuck into unvarying quick beats which would accelerate even further. Though it was mostly beyond her capability to impose any intellectual control on her playing her physical and emotional involvement with it was complete. My job at first was to catch this playing and make musical contact so she could at least have the experience of playing together with someone. Gradually I began to put this same quick beat into different musical contexts: playing with every beat, then playing a slow accompaniment against her fast beat; playing in 3/4 time; phrasing strongly; playing episodically against her continuity. This was never to contradict but to give her a different musical experience of what at the time was the only way she could play [⊙3]. I made use of one of music's major gifts – being able to say different things at the same time without it being a contradiction. This also continually emphasised the living, responsive nature of the musical relationship, of which she became increasingly aware, shooting me occasional quick glances of glee. Her face changed when she was playing music – it looked even younger, but also free, light and joyous.

Progress was incredibly slow, yet at the same time our music-making was never simply a replay of the previous week – there was always some small musical gain: in getting around habitual patterns or in an awareness of our togetherness in the music, perceptible in slight adjustments of tempo to each other's playing. We often both vocalised as we played, and I found this a good way to bring our playing back together when Em's drumming began to run away with itself. A song developed out of an improvisation: 'Emanuella, Emanuella, she can play the drum very well...', which Em would sing whilst accompanying herself on the drum [⊙4]. Occasionally she would also burst into (I presume) a Yiddish song, raise her arms in the air and dance in the chair. The way in which music obviously tapped into memories of her past and her culture was just another aspect of how music 'quickened' Em, how it freed the joy and life in her from the constriction of the fear and ritual that usually dominated her life.

> 'That was great Em, how about playing the cymbal now?'
>
> 'No! No! *NO!*...yes.'

The 'yes' was said as if in brackets, softly in an aside. I got used to this with Em – she would often say 'no' on principle, but if you listened to the quiet voice afterwards this often told you what she really wanted. Em was, perhaps, like many of us, genuinely frightened of what she wanted and encased herself in her own habit of rejection. To the last session I did with Em, two-and-a-half years from the first, I still got a rough reception. But I was also aware that she knew exactly why I was coming, talked about it for hours before and was disappointed when I could not come. At first I underestimated her sense of time, and turned up unprepared on a Thursday afternoon instead of Friday once in order to deal with some mishap in my timetable. Em took one disgruntled look at me and said 'Go avay Gary! I will see you tomorrow, Friday.'

Em usually rejected overtures of a conventional conversation, even with people she knew well. But again the music freed her and, mid-way through an improvisation, she would often stop suddenly, hold her drumstick up in the air and announce to me something which had presumably been on her mind. These comments were mostly about the people in her life, but on occasion the Chief Rabbi and others featured as well. This further demonstrated the fact that Em was more concretely involved with her life, intellectually and emotionally, than some people would have liked to believe.

Em's main instrument was the drum, but she would also play for a short time on a cymbal, and on some chime bars. Again her playing was simple but involved. Unlike some of the case studies in this book, with Emanuella there was no dramatic musical development, as indeed there was no dramatic personal development. 'Development' is often used as the criteria for the worth of a therapy, yet it is simply the wrong criteria to judge the work in this instance. As our opening script remained constant so, to an extent, did our music-making during the time we worked together. Em found something new (I like to think perhaps a measure of freedom) not by going beyond her limitations, but by somehow expanding within them. In the same way as I would take the only way she could play music and put it into different musical contexts, so she perhaps found in our creative musical relationship a new sense of herself *within* her limits. The essence of the process with Em was not a development from week to week but the weekly transformation that happened 'while the music lasts'. Rather than her circle of habit becoming necessarily any larger it perhaps became instead a dotted line – not so rigid and impervious to anything or anybody making contact.

Em was always clear when she had had enough, suddenly announcing:

> 'Thank you very much Gary!'
>
> 'Thank you, Em. That was lovely playing.'
>
> 'OK.'

We always finished with a goodbye song, and here there was always a genuine musical dialogue between us – an equal sharing of the music. The song had spaces in it to sing each others name, and Em sang her own name with satisfaction, but was rather inclined to forget me [⊙5]. Despite this, there were very few occasions when we both did not feel substantially better after the music. These sessions would be the few I would be sorely tempted to use 'before and after' photographs in response to the calls for justification for the effectiveness of music therapy. Em always looked qualitatively better in a dramatic way. Before she was usually tense, defensive and often aggressive. After, her face had softened and she seemed both pleased and comfortable with herself. Sometimes she would reach over and softly stroke the side of my cheek with her hand:

'I love you darlink...'

'I love you too, Em.'

LISTENING GUIDE

[⊙1] Em sits on a sofa which is about four yards from where the therapist sits at the piano. He sings hello to her with a song which is repeated each week. The song has enough spaces in it for Em to join in, and her curt rebuttals make a curious dialogue with the therapist's singing.

[⊙2] The therapist plays music in a quickish tempo. Em, who still sits on the sofa, joins in after a short time by clapping to the music (this can just be heard in the background). The therapist slows down his playing when she stops, then takes her tempo when she starts clapping again (this time louder). After a while she stops again and says 'that's enough!'. The therapist replies by singing back 'come and play the drum Emanuella!', to which she says 'No, I don't want to play the drum!' To encourage her the therapist starts to play the drum himself (it is placed just at the upper keyboard of the piano, and he plays with his right hand, continuing to play the piano with the left). Em starts clapping again and the therapist matches his piano/drum to her claps. When this also dies down he again sings 'Emanuella!', which provokes from her first an angry loud 'STOP IT! but then (with the rolled-up *Jewish Chronicle* on the coffee table) loud metrical slaps which become part of the music. Both Em and the therapist musically react to each other in a small structure which even includes Em's 'No' at the end...

[⊙3] Em now sits in a chair near the piano with the drum in front of her and a single drumstick in her hand. The piano plays at first, encouraging Em to start playing. When she does begin she plays in short bursts. The therapist sings along with the playing to encourage continuity in her playing.

[ω4] The song *Emanuella, Emanuella, she can play the drum very well...* had been developed in the course of previous sessions and it serves to reorientate her playing or help her get out of a rut. She sings along herself as well.

[ω5] The goodbye song is also well known to Em, and she sings it with obvious pleasure. She now sits at the piano, to the right side of the therapist. Towards the end of the excerpt you hear Em play the upper notes of the piano.

CHAPTER 6

Just a Minute...

> What is true of the human body is also true of the musical organism: its outward aspects are determined from within...the primal force, once it has initiated the motion, will strive spontaneously to sustain its life, taking on a momentum until it realises itself fully, like any other form of nature. (Heinrich Schenker)

God resides in the details, said Cézanne. The problem, however, in writing case studies such as the one preceeding is that much detail is inevitably lost. During the time we worked together Emanuella and I played perhaps a hundred hours of music, yet in the case study the process must be characterised in generalisations coupled with the specifics of a few dramatic incidents. This is inevitable of course, and a music therapy case study can no more be a blow-by-blow account of every single second of the music than can an autobiography be of every minute of a life. Yet in Creative Music Therapy what happens inside each minute is both the essence of this process, and a microcosm of larger trends. The detail shows the qualities and tendencies of the client's playing, the quality of the musical relationship between therapist and client, and demonstrates the potential or problems for further development in the therapy.

LISTENING BACK

In improvisation seconds count – the purely musical method of Creative Music Therapy lies in the detailed work which happens within the creative musical relationship in improvisation. It is not just a luxury that the therapist tapes every session, and listens back to as many as possible. Indeed Paul Nordoff stated that this work would not have been possible before the invention of the tape recorder. Because both therapist and client are playing together in the session it is difficult for the therapist to hear objectively – she herself is part of what happens, and memories are simply not powerful or reliable enough to remember even five minutes of music in any detail. Consequently a re-hearing of the session on tape later can be very necessary in finding out more objectively what 'really' happened in the session. The therapist is listening not just to what the music was, but *how* it was played: how the client plays music (what are the qualities and tendencies of his playing) and how the client and therapist are interacting with each other in the music. The therapist also listens to whether what she was actually doing matched her intentions – was she doing what she thought she was doing? What are her aims and possible strategies for the next session and, looking further, what are the longer term therapeutic aims for this client?

What follows in this chapter is a detailed version of the analytic re-hearing a therapist might make. More usually she will perhaps listen to the session as a whole quite quickly but concentrating in detail on particularly interesting passages. Many therapists working in the tradition of Creative Music Therapy write this process in note form (what we call an 'index sheet'), correlating observations against the numbers of the tape recorder. The example which follows is a very detailed version of this process, attempting to illustrate both what is happening, almost second by second in the music, and how this shows a method of music therapy in action. No working therapist could go into this detail of course (two minutes of musical time took me approximately eight hours to transcribe and annotate). An experienced therapist will, however, be working to much the same principle: whether this is written 'short-hand' or simply an intuitive hearing bolstered by experience.

The following is, then, the 'long-hand' version, for which I have also provided a transcription of the music (see Figure 6.1). The commentary on the music is given in the form of an 'index sheet': divided into two columns representing the two players – therapist and client (see Table 6.1). It attempts to describe not just what happened, but *how* and, to some extent, 'why'. The first question describes the music itself; the second the qualities and tendencies of the client's and therapist's playing (i.e. *how* they play what they play); the third suggests 'reasons' for any of the therapist's strategies or the client's reactions (though these are mostly limited to musical ones).

The episode illustrated in Figure 6.1 and Table 6.1 is described in 'A Detailed Example' (pp.55–56).

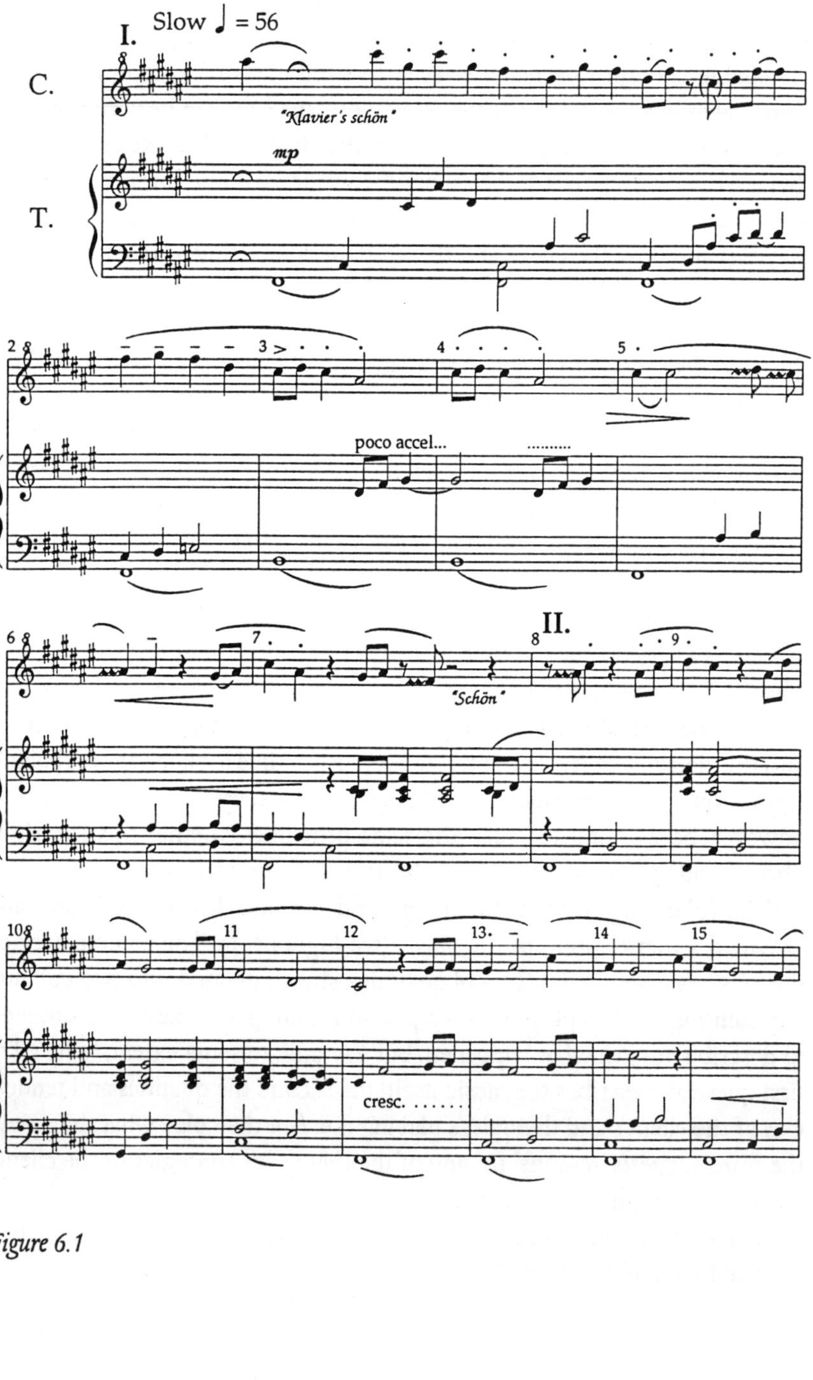

Figure 6.1

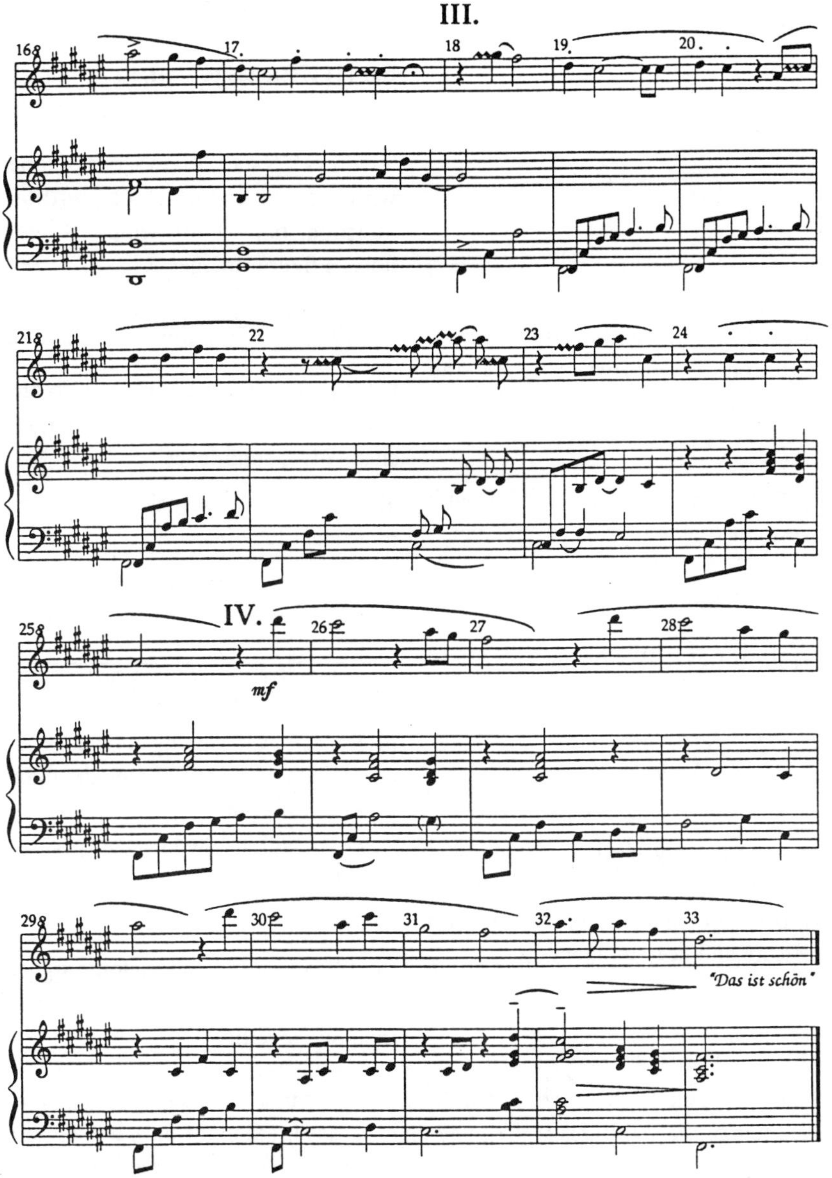

Figure 6.1 (continued)

Table 6.1

THERAPIST	**CLIENT**
	Bar [1] Hesitates to start.
Bar [1] Plays bass note of root chord.	
	Shadows T.'s start. Plays series of tones which seem unconnected, without direction, but set the tempo. After 8 notes a figure emerges… (i) 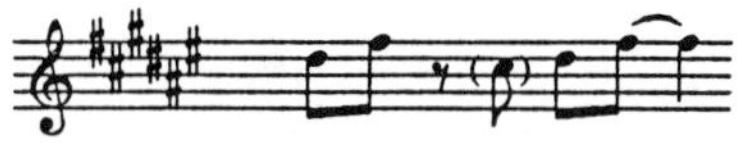
Picks figure (i) up and both repeat it together. T. reinforces figure and demonstrates 'I'm listening.'	[2] Plays a melodic phrase. Notes connect and lead somewhere. Emerging shape gives confidence.
[2] Encourages melodic direction with harmonic 'pull' in $F^{\#}$–B progression.	T. and C. feeling the melodic-harmonic movement together.
	[3] 4/4 metre established. New melodic figure emerges… (ii) 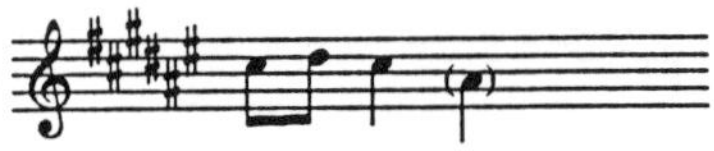
[3] Imitates (ii) rhythmically and melodically in inversion. (iii) 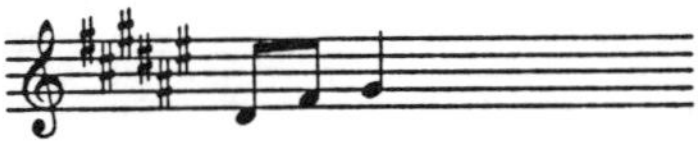	[4] Repeats ex.ii: gaining coherence and confidence. Variation of melodic figure with a different rhythm…ends [5], however, with marked hesitation & loss of stability.
[5]–[7] Supporting harmonically the growing melody. Hearing instability of C. in [5] strong bass note at beginning of bar and imitation of figure helps reassure and keep momentum.	[6]–[7] series of small melodic figures related to each other. C. and T. play the final one together.

T. and C. begin to share *intention* in the music, i.e. think together musically, make the same musical gestures at the same time. Not as in 'thought out', but a letting the logic of the music play itself. This produces a feeling of musical contact between T. and C.

Hears hesitation in melody: harmonically confirms tonic cadence.	[7] Brings phrase to tonic cadence, hesitates before final note (tonic $F^{\#}$). But it feels right. She says 'beautiful!'

THERAPIST

II

[7]–[8] Hears C. possibly losing continuity after cadence. Encourages continuation by repeating cadential motif over bar...

(iv) 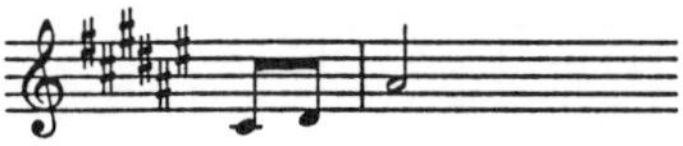

CLIENT

[8] Follows T., playing A# late (the 'arrival note' of T.'s phrase)

(v) 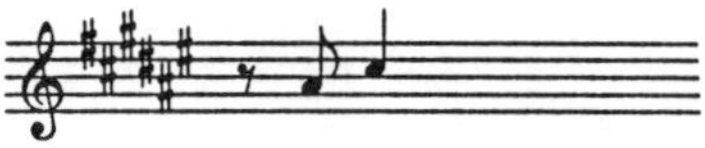

[8]–[19] Second section of piece as a whole. Demonstrates some sense of an overall shape, not just a bar-by-bar progression.

§ C.'s playing finding:

- melodic/rhythmic coherence and confidence;
- shape and direction;
- awareness of playing creatively with T.

Once C. is playing again T. retreats, allowing her to take melodic initiative. Supports with harmonic rhythm...

(vi) 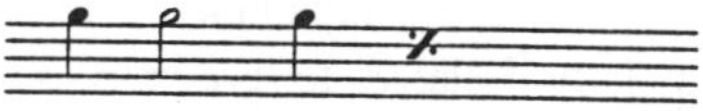

[12] T. initiates overlapping cadence with motif based on (ii), again to keep momentum going...

[8]–[12] Long melodic phrase made of related motifs, basically...

(vii) 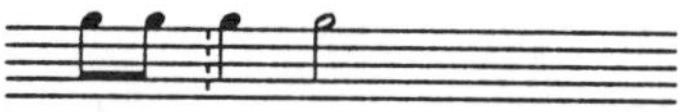

Phrase gracefully cadences at [12] Tendency to lose initiative at cadences.

Picks up T.'s motif mid-way and both play the second half of it together...

(viii) 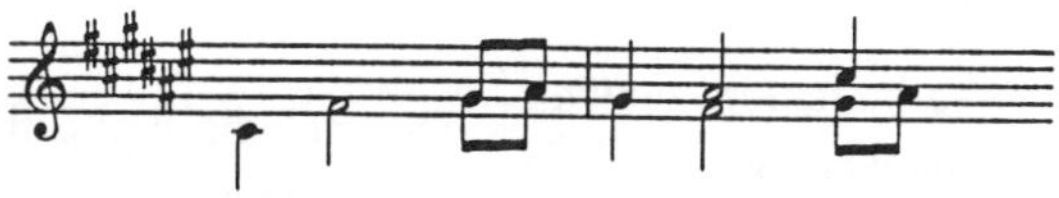

*T. and C. begin at the end of this bar to play in counterpoint – the natural musical device of playing the same musical idea in a 'different' way. They both hear and feel they are now really playing *together* in an inventive way.

[13]–[14] 3-bar phrase gets melodically limited. Loses direction.

THERAPIST | **CLIENT**

[14]–[15] Provides harmonic tension to help 'direct' C.'s melody.

Picks up harmonic tension and reacts to it…

[16] Unexpected exciting melodic leap of 10th, then phrased down…

(ix) 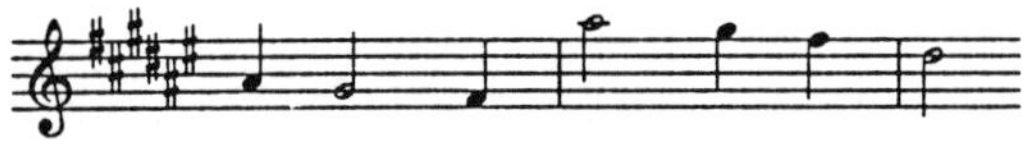

Supports with strong harmonic shift

[17] Feels implicit cadence but hesitates and loses way…

T. intervenes and takes the initiative melodically, also securing cadence at [18] with strong tonic bass.

Picks up T.'s cadence and plays cadential figure…

(x) 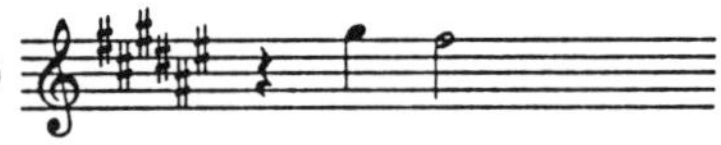

§ Confidence to 'take a leap' alternating with hesitation and lack of impulse for continuity.

III

[19] Sensing loss of confidence and momentum initiates a stronger accompaniment figure in bass – gives sense of forward movement without taking over melodic responsibility.

(xi) 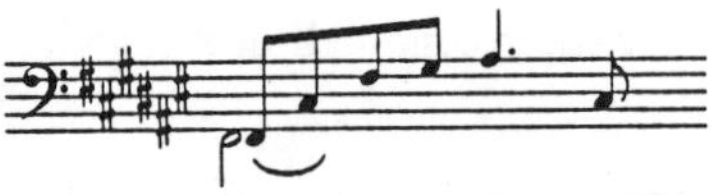

[19] Starts more confidently with T.'s supporting accompaniment. Finds new melody (related to previous motifs). Strong relationship between melody and accompaniment:

Nearly extends melody to a balanced 4-bar phrase, but hesitates and loses confidence in final bar.

In [22] T. reacts to hesitation, slowing down accompaniment and starting [23] with strong down-beat, emphasising rhythm…

(xii) 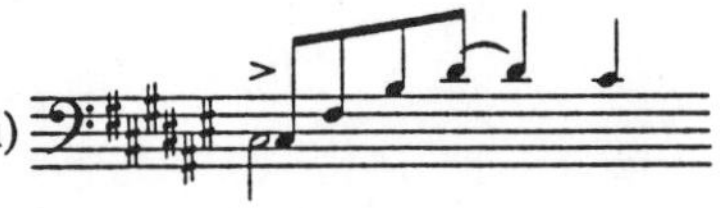

The melodic figure that was hesitant and incoherent at end of [22] restated with confident rhythm – as result of T.'s impulse. T. and C. share the shape of phrase in [23].

(xiii) 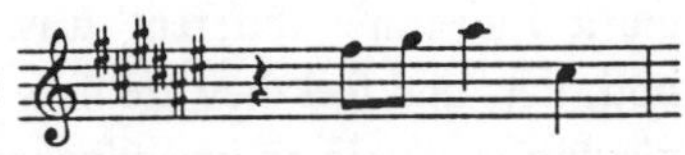

[24] Again sensing loss of impetus from C., T. plays stronger harmony with quaver movement in bass. Intensifying.

Keeps going and makes successful melodic cadence in [25].

THERAPIST	CLIENT
IV [26]–[31] Supports C.'s melody with harmonic rhythm and arpeggiated bass to keep momentum going.	[25]–[26] Initiates another new melodic impetus. Related to previous motifs. This time extends into a perfectly balanced melodic phrase of 8 bars: [26]–[33]

(xiv)

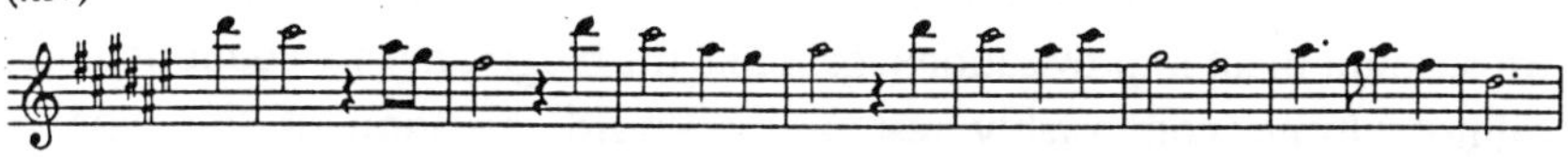

T. and C. share the sense and direction of the music. Mutual listening is demonstrated in motifs echoed or exchanged (e.g. [26]–[27]). [31] T. imitates strongly the motif and points out the inevitable cadence.	C.'s playing has shape and direction, she finds initiative and confidence. Cadences the melody with certainty. Says 'that was beautiful'.

This method shares some, but not all, of the characteristics of how a musicologist might analyse, say, a Mozart symphony. Both attempt to explain something about musical process from hindsight. But whilst the music analyst asks, what happens to this melody? the therapist asks, *how* does this person play this melody? or perhaps even, how is this person 'as' melody? The music analyst works with completed compositions notated as a text, whereas the therapist is listening directly to a person-in-the-music, a living improvised musical dialogue between two people.

A DETAILED EXAMPLE

The example I chose is a two-minute episode which, though short, is complete in itself and both simple and clear. It came from a first session with a non-impaired adult client with a chronic illness. She had no musical training, was very intimidated at playing anything and disliked the percussion instruments. Her playing on a drum tended to be very tentative, fragmented and uncertain: it had no sense of continuity or flow and I felt that all the music and initiative came from me. I asked her whether she would like to play the piano with me instead and she seemed much happier. We played the piano as a duet, with her at the treble end of the keyboard. She was still frightened of playing and I suggested that, to make it even simpler, she play with one finger on the black notes only. She was very nervous at first, but at the end of this two-minute piece was pleased with herself. When she left the hospital a few weeks later she said it was this two minutes on the piano that she remembered more than anything else [⊙6]. The transcription of this is given in Figure 6.1 (pp.50–51).

MUSICALLY GROUNDED INFERENCES

Such an analysis must to some extent be an interpretation of what happened. An account of an improvisation (again like the biographer's account of a life) cannot always comfortably rest on backward causation of the type 'x happened because of y, which led to z'. Improvising music together is a situation where some events seemingly happen simultaneously rather than obviously causing each other. In music this is actually quite common – a sharing of intention which is carried by the logic of the music rather than the separate decisions of the players.

Yet the account presented here as to what happened in the improvisation is very different from a psychodynamic-style interpretation, where a musical event is taken to have an extra-musical meaning. In the approach taken by Creative Music Therapy the therapist admittedly often needs to go beyond simple musical description in order to account for what happened in the improvisation. Nevertheless this is mostly at the level of what I call 'musically grounded inferences': that is, inferences whose musical basis can be intersubjectively validated by other listeners.

OUTWARD ASPECTS, INNER FORM

In the passage quoted as the epigraph to this chapter, the music analyst Heinrich Schenker compares a piece of music to a living organism. It seems to have, he writes, a momentum determined from some inner force which sustains its life and takes it through a process of growth until it has fulfilled itself. When the music is being improvised the metaphor seems even more apt. Here one can literally hear something grow from nothing and that 'its outward aspects are determined from within' (Schenker 1956). In the two minutes of music therapy looked at in this chapter this is true in two ways. First, in how the music seems to grow itself *between* the playing of the two people, pursuing not only their intentions but also its own. Second, there is also the sense in which the 'inner aspects' of the client's condition – her abilities, feeling and thoughts, influenced the 'outward aspects' of her playing. To an extent the therapist's intentions and musical actions are an attempt to moderate the negative aspects of these and foster the positive ones, so that the 'natural' process of musical invention, development and communication can happen between the therapist and client in the music. In the same format as the analysis, I summarise below in Table 6.2 what I think happened in the two minutes in more general terms.

Table 6.2

What is the therapist doing?	*What is the client doing?*
Creating musical meaning in dialogue with C.	Creating musical meaning in dialogue with T.
Supporting C.'s tentative finding of musical order and development by: stabilising; extending; sometimes echoing and developing C.'s musical gestures.	
T.'s listening is responsive and constructive.	Discovering 'on the spot' how the musical unfolding is shared by her and T. Feels listened to and that she is being musically understood.
Intervenes strongly only when necessary: to give direction, support, etc.	Feels supported and helped when hesitant and where the music seems to lose coherence.

Listening to the excerpt on the CD you hear two people playing, but often with the sense of there being only *one* music. The music therapy experience is based on this basic fact: of two or more people communicating musically as they experience both the music unfolding on its own natural path of growth whilst at the same time representing the expressive and communicative gestures of the players.

A final sense in which music resembles a living organism (a higher one, at least) is in the sense that the journey of its unfolding and development is not totally determined. To an extent it finds what it is doing, and where it is going, along the road it travels. The order governing a musical improvisation is found by the players *within* the actual unfolding of the music. The meaning of the journey is part of the travelling and the end-point is found only by virtue of the form completing itself.

All the characteristics of the music therapy process which happened in the microcosm of two minutes of a first session also happen on a larger scale. I hope that the remaining case studies in this book will show that, while based on the bedrock of the kind of detailed work shown in this chapter, there are also larger processes operating over the weeks, months and possibly years of work with a client, which are nevertheless similar in kind. The processes of musical invention, growth and development, support and communication shared between two people improvising music together are central to the music therapy process and are embedded in both the seconds and the years of the work.

CHAPTER 7

Herr G.

> The music was exquisite. The first time I didn't recognise it as a voice, but as some kind of mediaeval wind instrument. But the second time I knew it was a voice, that there was a person there, there was someone who didn't want to kill me.

Herr G. lay in a coma in the intensive care unit of a large hospital, his passivity contrasting with the activity and noise of the machines and the bright lights of the ward. Anyone who came into contact with him wore green surgical gowns and masks.

After a month in a coma he seemed to be dying, but nobody could account for the sudden decline in his state in the last few days. The doctors, his wife and daughters described for me the events that had led to this point. Herr G. was a successful businessman whose life, and the life of his family, revolved around work. His one hobby was travelling, he never listened to music but did have an obsession with the news, which he kept up with at least three times a day. His problems had begun two years earlier, culminating in a cardiac arrest. A month later, after a second attack, he had to be reanimated and was given a bypass operation. This was followed by kidney failure and thrombosis of the lungs. In July 1990 he had a heart transplant, after which he first recovered but then fell into a coma. He had made no reaction to anyone for one month and had been assessed as '3' on the Glasgow Coma Scale, indicating no response to auditory stimulus or pain.

A large man, he was now gaunt and collapsed and seemed really to be suffering. I asked the staff whether I could be alone with him for a short

---

Herr G. worked with Dr Dagmar Gustorff. She is joint-director of the Institut für Musiktherapie at the University of Witten-Herdecke, Germany. She wrote her doctoral thesis on the use of music therapy with coma patients, and the above case came from her work in the intensive care unit of the University Clinic, Münster.

time and if, after the music therapy session, they could leave him quietly without medical procedures for as long as possible. I talked to him quietly, explaining who I was and what I would do: that if he wanted I would just sing to him for a short while.

The first time I sang to him Herr G. turned his head towards me and, without moving or opening his eyes, seemed to be listening. At the end of the session, which was about six minutes, he also seemed to express in his gestures something like 'thank-you'.

During the thirteen sessions we had together there was just one musical motif, which came from a hymn. Though it became slightly more developed it remained essentially simple: a single phrase of unharmonised melody in d-minor. This may seem rather 'thin' to anyone else, but I came to realise how important it was not to do too much with a person in a coma who is both physically weak and mentally disorientated. The music has to be scaled down to their cognitive and emotional capacity. Families of other coma patients I have worked with have brought in radios or tapes with the idea that their relative will want music they are familiar with. Many patients have rejected this by shaking their head, but have indicated that they *do* want to be sung to. A Rachmaninov symphony is simply too potent: in the physical impact of the sound, in the concentration demanded to listen to it, not to mention the emotional strength. Rather like a medication, the quality and potency of the music must match the condition of the patient.

In contrast to pre-recorded music, coma patients including Herr G. have subsequently said that they felt the singing to be *their* music, intimately related to them. Certainly my starting-point is them, in the very basic sense that I take their breathing rhythm as the basis of the music. By entraining my singing with their fundamental rhythms (pulse and breathing) I can come alongside the only aspect of action and identity that a person has in this condition. For the time of the session it is not just a machine maintaining their breathing, but a person 'in sympathy' with it. If I were just breathing in time with him this would be a sharing of rhythm, but it is *melody* which adds the uniquely musical and therefore human element. Even a small melodic motif, repeated both within and between sessions, is something for the patient to make sense of, to remember, to identify with as his or her music. A person in a coma who has perhaps lost much of the cognitive capacity to process verbal language seems to be able to make sense of musical material – but only if it bears some relationship to them, and is of the right complexity.

The musical motif I sing and repeat for a person is something that is simple enough to be grasped as a whole and remembered. This is in stark contrast to the rest of the acoustic environment for a patient in intensive care, dominated by the random, meaningless and inhuman noise of machinery.

After one month of not reacting to anyone or anything, Herr G. made his first reaction during the singing. During the first four sessions I kept the music the same – a slow tempo with clear phrasing of the short melodic motif.

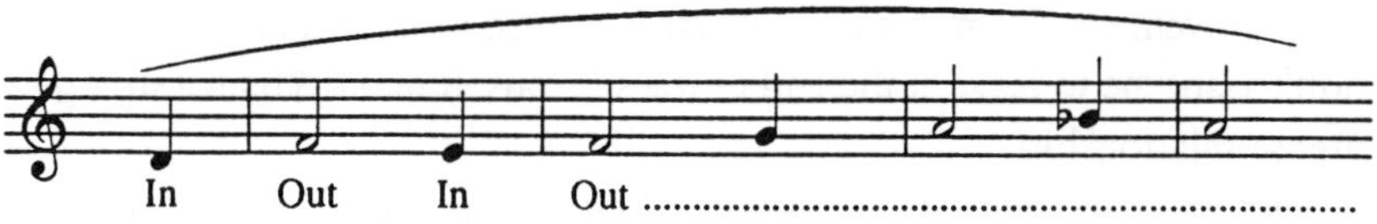

Figure 7.1

The phrasing was vital in that it included the breathing rhythms of both Herr G. and myself woven into the shape of the melody. Even in the early sessions there were almost imperceptible irregularities in Herr G.'s breathing unique to the period of the singing, which seemed to relate to the phrasing of the music. I felt it almost as a test from him – 'will she go with me?'

This was clarified in the fourth session when he clearly began breathing in phrases. By this I mean that at the end of the melodic phrase, when there is a short pause while I breathe, Herr G. would hold his breath slightly, listen and resume breathing when I sang again. This was the beginning of both a musical and a personal contact, of dialogue as quite literally a 'taking part' in the only way he could.

In an effort to get a reaction out of comatose patients I noticed that everyone – doctors, nurses, family – tended to shout orders: 'Open your eyes!', 'Can you hear me?'. In an attempt to be understood we often forget that how we communicate is more important than what we communicate, and that this is dependent on rhythm and inflection rather than volume.

Herr G. remained at level 3 of the Glasgow Coma Scale. At this time his wife was finding it very difficult to accept her husband's condition. The strong, capable man she knew formerly was now weak, helpless and passive. She was still, however, half expecting him to be effective, and was also putting the staff in the unit under a lot of strain to do something. The doctor asked me if she could be with us in the next music therapy session. She came and found that, despite her fears, there *was* still a person there, and that he could be reached. She cried afterwards, and we talked about how she could find her own way of making a contact with him.

In the next session one of his daughters also came to the session, and for the first time he held eye contact with me for a while. From this point onwards, at the request of both the doctors and the family, we made videos of subsequent sessions.

It was still not known whether Herr G. was paralysed, but in the seventh session he grasped my hand when I sang to him, and the next time also moved the left hand in a way that was obviously intentional rather than a reflex movement. From this time onwards he also made it quite clear that he didn't want me to leave at the end of the sessions. It had become a strangely intense relationship.

Paradoxically, during this period when his consciousness returned his body became weaker and again his hold on life seemed tenuous. Still his only significant form of response was during our sessions together. Perhaps inevitably, the staff seemed just a little defensive about the fact that the only positive signs with Herr G. came not from the copious efforts of high-tech medicine but from the work of a visiting music therapist who 'just' sang! They asked me none the less for advice, and I repeated what I had told Herr G.'s wife: that they should not keep demanding response, testing him, but instead ask him to help them, and to ask this softly, kindly and clearly. After this the nurses in particular started to copy my style of approach and contact. They stopped shouting, and touched him in a different way, not only for practical reasons, but touching him and talking to him 'just' for contact. Through what they saw happening in the music therapy sessions they had more faith in the reality of this person so seemingly inaccessible.

Before the tenth session I met Herr G.'s wife coming out of the room. 'I've just told him that you were coming and he seemed almost to smile' she said. When I went in and said hello he really did smile!

From the eleventh session onwards he was increasingly awake. He could indicate his needs now with gestures, but still couldn't even attempt to speak because of a tube in his mouth. He now clearly took part in the music, both phrasing his breathing and conducting with his arms. His face showed concentration and pleasure. In the twelfth session Herr G. took my hand and put it in the middle of my upper chest. It was Friday, and I had the feeling this would be the last time we would work this way.

This proved right. Monday morning I found him sitting up in bed. He smiled and nodded hello. He could now read his letters, write questions and answers and, characteristically (to his old self at least), had asked for the latest on the Dow-Jones Index! The work we had done before seemed inappropriate now, and that day we just talked. I told him my project was nearly completed and I would be leaving the hospital in the next few days. I felt, however, that we still needed a purely musical 'resolution' to our relationship, when we could play and not talk.

The next day I brought in a small pentatonic lyre which Herr G. sat up and played while I sang. It worked well, and we reached a point of shared music-making in that last session. Before he left the hospital some weeks later Herr G. had an interview with a psychologist and revealed some fascinating information which seemingly belies many of our assumptions about the experiential world of a person in a coma:

> After the operation I found myself on a battlefield in the Middle Ages. It was after the battle and my wife and some other soldiers wanted me dead – they were searching the battlefield for those still alive, and they meant to kill them. I felt I should die.
>
> The point it all changed was when I first heard the music. The music was exquisite! The first time I didn't recognise it as a voice, but as some kind of mediaeval wind instrument. But the second time I knew it was a voice, that there was a person there, there was someone who didn't want to kill me. I remember thinking, there *is* life, there is something else but this, there is someone who wants me to survive...and not only wants me, but is helping me to connect to life again.
>
> But every time people shouted at me I went back to the idea of dying. It was such a struggle to do anything, and when they shouted at me 'Open your eyes!' ten times a day I thought 'I'm not in the circus!'. I *decided* not to respond, or at least not to respond in those ways. The machines in the room I felt were bombs and weapons. But the music I felt was *my* music. I decided to live when I first heard the music...

It is known that people in a coma often experience quasi-psychotic states, which might explain Herr G.'s battlefield delusions. But equally, is his interpretation not understandable given the situation he found himself in? In coma a person is profoundly disorientated in both time and space, struggling to re-knit the connection between their inner and outer worlds. The environment of an intensive care unit does little to allay the fear, disorientation and alienation of the patient. In fact, the noise of the machines and the lack of intimate contact all too accurately fit Herr G.'s vision of being assaulted, of everything being hard and frightening, encouraging him to escape even by dying.

The singing, in contrast, was the only soft, personal element in his experience. It was the only contact which related to him as he was then (the only way he *could* be then), not demanding that he should be something else, something more. He felt it as his music, as a meeting in the music with another person on both a physical and an emotional level. With no speech, and little movement at first, this was the *only* way he could really experience someone being with him and accompanying him. It was the only way he could share something with another person, to take part, rather than be totally passive. But perhaps most of all he experienced the music as a call back to life.

Herr G. is now well again and back to work. He offers to come to talks I give on music therapy to tell his own story, and sends me a huge bouquet of flowers every Christmas!

The only unfortunate outcome was that a while ago a German tabloid newspaper got hold of the story and misrepresented it as a 'miracle'. What was really the miracle, however, was that we found a way of establishing musical contact and that music was the only thing that could carry the message to him – 'Live!'

LISTENING GUIDE

[⏻7] The short excerpt is taken from the soundtrack of one of the video recordings of Herr G.'s sessions. Though it is necessary to see the video to appreciate how he reacts, just listening nevertheless conveys the atmosphere this work took place in, and the dramatic contrast between the random noise of the machinery and the quiet intensity of the sung melody.

CHAPTER 8

Meeting

> All real living is meeting. Meeting is not in time and space, but space and time in meeting. (Martin Buber)

In Wagner's opera *The Flying Dutchman* the love duet between Senta and the Dutchman begins minutes after they have set eyes on each other for the first time. A clever direction in a recent production at Covent Garden had the lovers remain on opposite sides of the stage to sing their passionate duet, a situation which emphasised the extreme intimacy you can hear between them despite the fact they are strangers to each other.

A comparison of this scenario with the situation of the preceding case study may not be as fanciful as it may at first seem. In Herr G.'s case music also worked to create an unlikely contact between two people, even though he was not even conscious for much of the time of the therapy. From his own account it was clear that central to his experience of music therapy was the intimate, responsive relationship *inside* the music. In his condition this musical contact was the only way he could actively experience someone being with him. It was in this sense both a musical and a personal contact, which led to moments of what I shall call in this chapter 'musical meeting'.

THE RELATIONSHIP IN THE MUSIC

The touchstone of Creative Music Therapy is the quality of the relationship *in* the music. This is also the most difficult aspect of the work to explain in words, though when it occurs (and is experienced live, seen or heard recorded) it can be recognised by most people directly and unequivocably.

To begin with a practical illustration of this I want to take an example from a video of a colleague's first session with a client suffering from chronic pain. She plays two drums and two cymbals and for most of the session has seemed uninvolved with both her own playing and with the music the therapist improvises on the piano. Though both people are playing instruments there seems little relationship between them in the music. Then, in the simplest and most natural way, a contact is established. She plays a careful, slow beat alternating between both of the drums (see Figure 8.1).

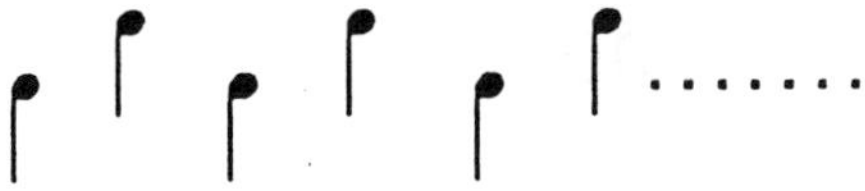

Figure 8.1

The therapist reduces the complexity of his music to just a simple rocking fifth in both hands (see Figure 8.2).

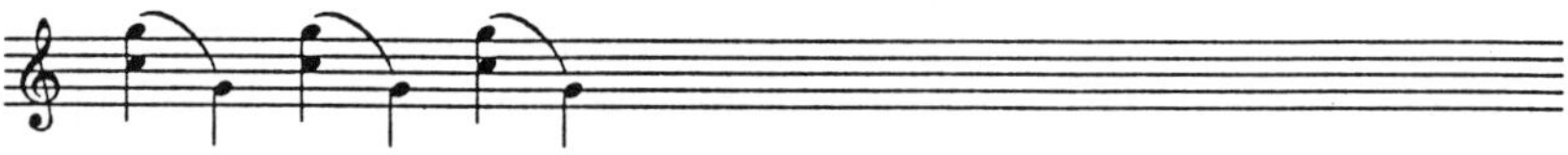

Figure 8.2

He matches this melodic figure to the time of her alternating drum-beats. It is not a direct mirroring, but a matching – an echo which also has a character and intent of its own. She hears this echo of her own playing and, probably for the first time in the session, experiences both her own playing in relation to the music as a whole and her relationship to the therapist *in the music.* The message that both are responding to each other is reinforced by slight changes of speed to which each then adjusts. In the penultimate beat a slight dissonance in the piano chord (caused by the B) gives a sense of the phrase resolving, and she in turn confirms this by carefully placing the next beat on the cymbal (see Figure 8.3).

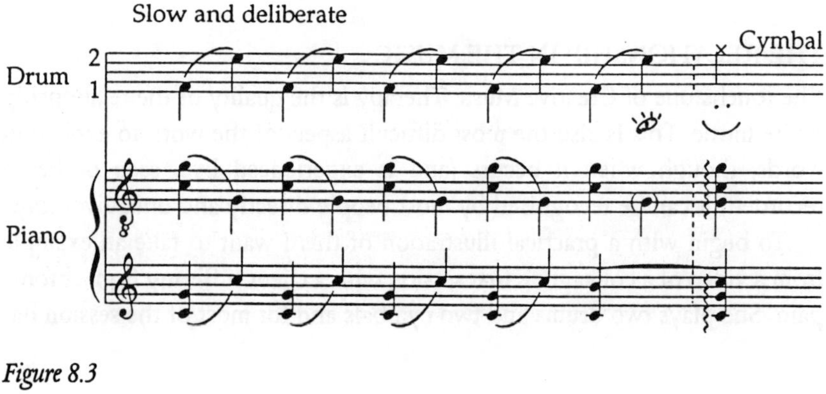

Figure 8.3

Just before she plays the cymbal she looks up towards the therapist and smiles as they play this last, inevitable beat together. This passage is a simple but nevertheless complete example of 'musical meeting', where both players share something of thought, feeling and intention within the purely musical.

MEETINGS

In several languages the word for 'meeting' can mean both something practical and something profound. The former concerns the everyday business of appointments negotiated in quantities of time and space. I might say 'I'll meet you at 6.00pm in front of the Festival Hall.' But we also use 'meeting' in the sense of a 'meeting of minds' or a 'meeting of hearts', states which are far from predictable or quantifiable.

It is this deeper form of meeting which the philosopher and theologian Martin Buber is referring to in the epigraph to this chapter.[1] Buber wrote much about the nature of dialogue and of the different qualities of relationships we have in our lives. In particular he brought attention to the difference between what he called 'I–it' relationships in contrast to the 'I–Thou' type: between a world to be used and a world to be 'met'. In the former the people or things we come into relationship with remain objects to us – to be experienced, used and manipulated. They always remain an 'It' to us and, though we may influence them, we do not allow them to influence us in return and therefore remain untouched by them. In comparison, it is possible to have a very different relationship with the world that confronts us – whether this be an object, a work of art, a person or God. In an 'I–Thou' relationship there is real 'meeting' within an intimate relationship, the outcome of which is that each side somehow changes the other, however subtly. These meetings take place not in the time of the clock or the space of the map but in a subjective world where there are unique qualities (rather than quantities) of time and space. Hence Buber's statement, 'meeting is not in space and time, but space and time in meeting' (Buber 1987). People talk, for example, of being 'lost' in the time of music, or prayer. And when we talk of being 'close' to someone we are not only meaning in terms of measurable physical space. It is difficult to quote Buber, since his ideas rely on an argument developed through an unusual vocabulary. In her book *The*

---

1 What I write here is no more than a suggestion of the implications of Buber's approach in reference to the particular form of dialogue that comes about in Creative Music Therapy. Buber's thought in all its complexity can be followed through in *I and Thou* and *The Way of Response*, a collection of his writings (Buber 1987 and 1966).

Quantum Self Danah Zohar, however, gives a clear account of the central idea:

> Intimacy is not a relationship between 'I' and 'You', or between 'I' and 'It', in which you or it (a book, a stone, a computer) influence *me*. In intimacy, I and you appear to influence *each other*, we seem to 'get inside' each other and change each other from within in such a way that 'I' and 'You' become a 'We'. This 'We' that we experience is not just 'I + You', it is a new thing in itself, a new entity...the 'We' that appears to arise in intimate relationships is the 'I-Thou' written about by Martin Buber. (Zohar 1990)

THE 'BETWEEN'

This 'We', the common ground where 'I–Thou' relationships can be forged, Buber called the 'Between'.[2] In music therapy the 'Between' is the music itself, where our creative responses can draw an 'I' and a 'You' into an 'I–You' and finally perhaps into 'We'. In comparison to listening to recorded music, where the hearer has no possibility of his response influencing the disc, improvising music with someone brings about quite naturally a situation of mutual response.

I remember struggling once to explain music therapy to somebody. After a while she said, 'I see – it's like the difference between being on land and being in water. Suddenly you feel different – freer, supported, you can do different things.' Changing the medium you are acting in, whether from land to water, or from words to music, can give a different feeling of both yourself and how you relate to other people. Within this 'musical between' a relationship can come about which is primarily *in* the music, established in the improvisation from the first time a musical contact is made, and developed through to the point where a true 'meeting' can come in the music.

FROM CONTACT TO MEETING IN THE MUSIC

In the music therapy situation the 'musical meeting' cannot happen until the client and therapist have made contact in the music. This is the therapist's first task – in Nordoff and Robbins' words 'to search out the region of

---

2 'that mode of existence I call "the between" or "between-ness". That is the mode of existence between persons communicating with one another, which we cannot co-ordinate with either the psychic or the physical realms... Leaping fire is indeed the right image for the dynamic between persons in "We"' (Buber 1966).

contact'. In *Therapy in Music for Handicapped Children* (1971) they describe how a musical relationship is established with a five-year-old psychotic child:

> The drum-beating was not at first a consciously self-directed activity for this boy. He was utterly absorbed in realising expression of the rhythmic impulses that lived within him. Consciousness of what he was doing developed later in the sessions as he experienced his beating impulses being answered in the music that surrounded him. When this happened, and the boy and I really met in the music, the activity that had been an unpredictable game began to take on the form of a musical give-and-take. (Nordoff and Robbins 1971)

The relationship comes, the musical meeting potentially happens, when the boy experiences something more than himself; when he experiences a relationship *between* his playing and the music of the therapist. He hears himself being heard and responds to his being responded to. Experience seems to show that the initial stages of music therapy often follow this same pattern of musical contact leading on to 'musical meeting' whoever the client (adult or child) and whatever their condition or level of conventional musical ability.

A SCHEMA OF MUSICAL RELATIONSHIP

The remainder of this chapter is a schematised illustration of the different levels of relationship possible between two (or more) players within a music therapy context. This must be prefaced, however, with some warnings, since no real client is either as simple or as clear as a schema seems to suggest. Moreover, the notion of a progression or development through the following situations can be misleading: since for every client who seems to follow a logical development there is another with whom no such logic exists. What looks like the goal of therapy, 'meeting', could (and indeed sometimes does) come not as a hard-won victory but naturally and immediately in the first minutes of playing together with someone. It is not, then, an inevitable progression from conditions 1–4: a client need neither begin at 1 nor attain 4. The schema should rather be seen as a possible logic of an approach (developed from many therapist's experience of Creative Music Therapy), into which individual clients can fit in a diversity of individual ways.

A possible initial situation is that a client plays in a first session (or continues to play) as if in a self-contained bubble. In contrast the music the therapist improvises on the piano is a close response to everything about the client – attempting to describe musically not just the character and quality of the playing, but also the physical and emotional aspects of the person in that moment. The playing closely 'accompanies' the client – both in the everyday sense of walking beside, but also as a musical accompanist plays with a singer, for example. It is not a direct mirroring, but a moving beside a person, a matching and echoing which nevertheless retains its own character, intent and musical meaning.

In this condition the client plays an instrument but may be substantially unaware that the therapist's playing relates to hers, or else not perceive the music as something separate from her own playing. We could represent it as a diagram (Figure 8.4), where the therapist is intentionally responding to the client's playing ('I'>'You'), but the client experiences only herself in the music ('I'):[3]

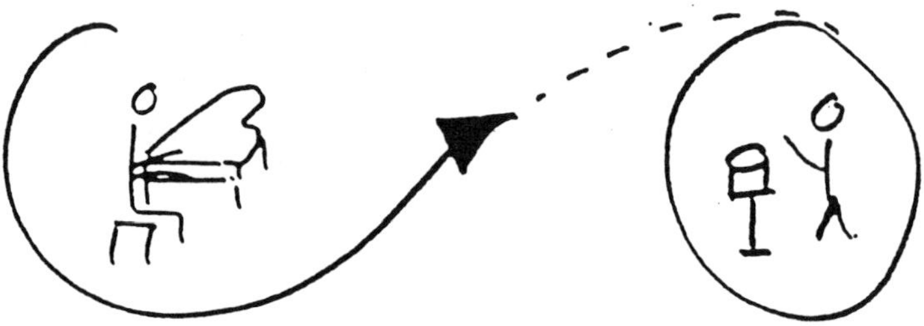

Figure 8.4 Contacting

The curved arrow shape going from the therapist to the client in Figure 8.4 represents the purely musical reaching out to contact. It need involve no eye contact. Equally the closed bubble around the client represents a *musical* isolation. This may, however, be accompanied by eye contact with the therapist and other social gestures.

A variation on this first situation is where a client is from the start fully aware of the therapist's music and 'shadows' it. This is more a form of reaction than a response since there is no real mutuality in which to meet musically (Figure 8.5).

---

3 There is, however, always *some* relation between two people playing music in the same room, even if this is mostly unconscious – as in the effect of background music. Here the client could be said to react rather than respond to the music.

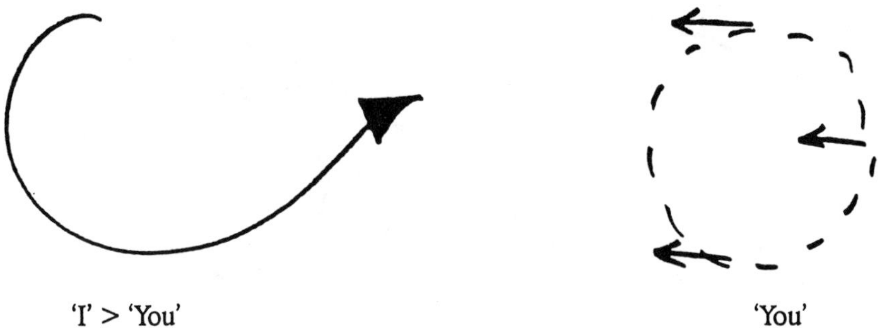

Figure 8.5

This is not to say that there is no musical contact or meeting unless the client is playing something. I can still improvise music to match the rocking of an autistic child or, in the case of work with unconscious patients, the therapist can entrain her singing to the primary rhythms of the patient's physiology. At first it is likely this situation will be the same as that of the person playing the drum with the therapist – the patient is unaware of the music that is 'accompanying' him. Equally, however, it can progress to a musical contact and even meeting as a sharing of response.

Contact happens when the client hears herself being heard.[4] Like the woman in the video described at the beginning of this chapter, there is a precise moment when the client hears that the music *includes* her, that she is being responded to in the music and can possibly respond back. The closed circle begins to open – musically 'I' becomes 'I' (You?) as in Figure 8.6.

The figure may make it seem that the therapist is somehow 'swallowing up' the client and his individuality or self-sufficiency. On the contrary, it is more a situation where both people begin to share one flow of musical experience. It is not so important who approached who first, but that mutual contact is made. In Herr G.'s case it was the way in which the therapist physically related the melody she sang to him which made a contact through the barrier of the coma. He first became conscious of being responded to *in* the music, and then from a point of contact he was able to share in the music by 'breathing in phrases' – which was a musical response in the only way

4 As Oliver Sacks writes: 'We see that the contactual is essentially musical, as the musical is essentially contactual... The touchless moving-together in an intuitive kinetic sympathy of attunement – this is genuine art...which can never be simulated by any mechanical feedback; for it is only an ever-changing, melodic and *living* play of forces which can recall living beings into their own living being' (Sacks 1991).

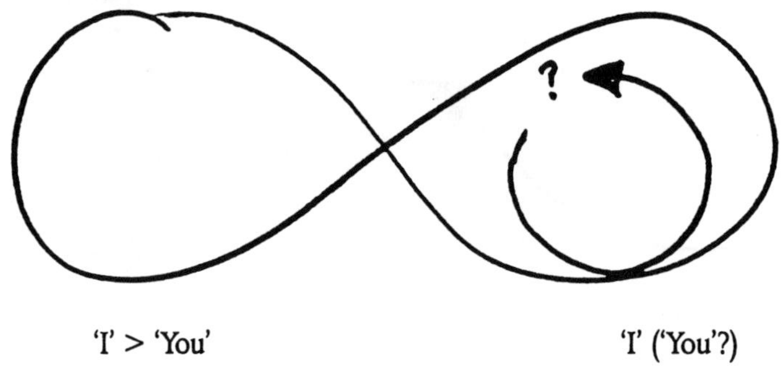

Figure 8.6 Responding

that was physically possible for him. This situation is not so different in principle as one might first suspect from a more conventional music therapy session, with the client actively playing an instrument.

When musical response has been established real communication is possible in the music. In this situation the client is aware of her own playing and how that playing relates to, and is answered by, the therapist's playing. She also finds out that what she intentionally plays affects the music as a whole – that she can influence the tempo, dynamics and character of the music. She finds that she can respond to the therapist's playing as well – that both can answer each other in the music and that this musical relationship can at the same time be a very satisfying human relationship, a feeling of being understood and accepted by someone else. The closed circle is further loosened as dialogue is established (Figure 8.7).

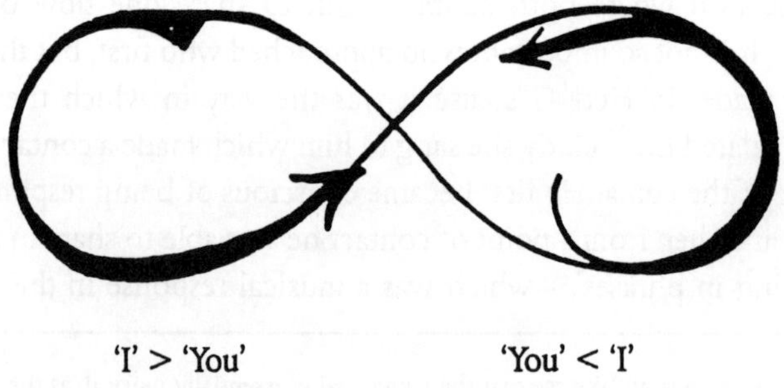

Figure 8.7 Relating

Here client and therapist enter into a genuine musical relationship. In dialogue they begin to create something together rather than just remaining two separate self-contained forces which, like colliding billiard-balls, effect each other without changing each other. On the contrary, musical dialogue is a flow of meaning between people which includes physical, emotional and intellectual experience. Dialogue in this sense allows a 'becoming together' rather than just a 'being together'.

This flow of musical meaning in dialogue lives partly in the intentional gestures both players make in response to each other. But it is more than just the alternating form of a verbal dialogue. In music both people play together and respond to each through the sense of the music itself – its rhythmic, melodic and harmonic 'necessities' – how, that is, tempo ebbs and flows; how rhythms 'want' to repeat and develop; how melodic phrases 'want' to complete themselves, and so on. For much of the time, in a way not intentionally directed by either player, the music takes them up and almost, you could say, plays them. Think of the very first example, where the client and therapist cadence the simple phrase, the therapist with a dissonant note resolving, the client with a cymbal stroke. At this point they shared intention in the music (or perhaps the music gave them a shared intention at that point in time). When there is a musical contact the players share the present: in the 'musical meeting' they also share something of the future (in where the music 'wants to go'). Here 'I–You' has become 'We' (Figure 8.8).

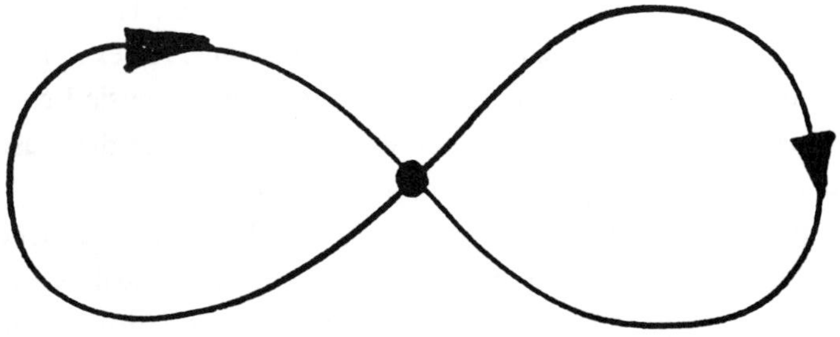

Figure 8.8 Meeting

The 'musical meeting' is not something vague, but happens at a specific 'meeting point' in the music. Hearing these points on the tape it is clear what is happening, and we can perhaps imagine what the experience of the people playing is like: when, for these instants, there is a unity of action, thinking and feeling.

Buber wrote that meeting is not in our everyday space and time, but that the meeting has its own qualities of space and time. The 'musical meeting' happens in the qualities of musical time and space, in a sense which is not just metaphor. At its simplest level music has its own time in its pulse and rhythm, and its own space in its melody and harmony. Meeting in the 'time' of the music is not as in a measured duration, but as a being-together in synchrony;[5] being in the 'space' of music is not as in a measured distance, but as a shared shape which has a direction towards the future. It makes little sense, however, to separate out these phenomena as each aspect influences all the others. Meeting cannot be forced or manufactured – it simply happens when the level of listening and consciousness is right and when the music acts like gravity, pulling the players into relationship. This can happen within the first minute of the first session, or not until the eleventh hour. Contact can be simultaneous with meeting or there can be a considerable wait between making musical contact and really meeting in the music.

THE EXPERIENCE OF 'MUSICAL MEETING'

When meeting does happen for the first time in a music therapy session it is often accompanied by a puzzled or a delighted smile, as it was with the woman in the video. As Francis said to music therapist Colin Lee, 'and when something musically happens and you smile, and I think it's beautiful, it works, it's there, and it was something that just happened'. The experience is not always comfortable. A client of another colleague, for example, said 'It's fascinating. When I think of expressing myself in the music I can hear only my own inner gesture coming out. But when I listen to the music it's terrifying, because I can hear the two of us meeting!'

Music therapists often work with people to whom the experience of intimacy in the musical meeting can be at odds with their usual experience of life: where their psychological, physical or social condition has led to isolation, to not being able to communicate well and having the feeling of 'missing' rather than meeting in relationships.

---

5 There is also sometimes the quality of a 'timeless moment' when people meet in the music. The Greeks used two terms for time: 'chronos', meaning passing time, and 'kairos' – 'a point of time filled with significance, charged with past and future, and instant of temporal integration' (Kermode 1967).

This same situation can be experienced by people who on the surface seem to have little in common. At the extreme end of the scale is the isolation of the autistic child with whom you can be in the same place and time but fail to find any conventional point of contact. It is perhaps easier for us to appreciate the situation of many adults with learning difficulties by comparing their problems with language to our own frustrating and isolating experiences in a foreign tongue. A barrier to meeting can be there in the same way, however, with someone intellectually skilled and verbally fluent. The reason for not being able to communicate as they would want may be difficult to find. It may be due to an underlying psychological problem or simply the fact that they have forgotten how to listen (to another person or to themselves), or believe that they are never fully heard by another person.[6]

The experience of meeting in the music can be a compensation to all these people in an intimacy which is not manufactured or forced but comes naturally out of the situation where two or more people can become one in the music.

Musical meeting comes and goes. It is never constant, as in everyday relationships intimacy is not constant. Buber stated that even when we achieve the 'I–Thou' relationship it will always fall back into 'I–It' again. In music, if we stop listening contact is lost, and along with this the possibility of musical meeting. Nevertheless the musical meeting once achieved is the starting-point and the constant touchstone for the development and maturing of the therapeutic relationship in Creative Music Therapy. Once the intimacy has been achieved there is a confidence between client and therapist which allows them to work with mutual creativity on the dialogue between their musical and personal worlds.

6 Though music therapists are generally cautious about suggesting explanations of these phenomena, there is some evidence linking problems of basic emotional and physiological self-organisation with the ability to attain or sustain any level of musical contact and inter-communication. See Chapter 15.

CHAPTER 9

Karl

The daring first notes of song
Pierced through the barren numbness... (Rilke)

As he sat in a wheelchair edging himself along, my first impression of Karl was of a man in slow motion. The occasional expressions on an otherwise blank face also seemed slowed down, and would freeze artificially on him. Yet he was still just twenty-five years old, with a strong, muscular body.

The terrible irony was that the beginning of his tragedy had started just five years ago as he ran at high speed around a field playing his favourite sport, American football. After some breathing difficulties while playing he consulted a doctor and his condition seemed to snowball from there. A problem was discovered in a major artery and Karl underwent several successful operations. Then, quite inexplicably, he had a heart attack whilst being transferred to another hospital and needed to be reanimated. It is not known exactly how long he was clinically dead, but the result of oxygen starvation during this period left him with severe neurological damage.

Karl ended up in intensive care, but later emerged alive though helpless – unable to move or speak. It only gradually emerged in the months that followed that, although tetraplegic, his intellectual functioning had by some miracle survived unimpaired. He soon began, and was remarkably successful in, a programme of physical rehabilitation. Movement was regained of a sort, but is was all painfully artificial in its quality – slow, intentional and effortful.

Speech and the ability to communicate were not returning, however. A speech therapist concluded that Karl would not be able to recover his speech as there seemed to be no voice there to work with. Instead he was given a

---

Karl's music therapist was Peter Hoffmann, who works at the Gemeinschaftskrankenhaus in Herdecke, West Germany – a general hospital for people with acute and chronic illness.

computer system to try to communicate with – a help, of course, but also to Karl yet another barrier between him and other people.

Karl came to me after having consulted a physiologist for a second opinion about his speech. The specialist could only confirm the earlier opinion of the speech therapist, that he was unlikely to develop speech consciously again. The doctor also saw, however, that Karl's current depression centred around his problem with communicating. He suggested music therapy and contacted me to ask if I could work with Karl.

This, then, was how I introduced music therapy to Karl – suggesting the link between music and communication, but being careful to add, 'I don't want to work directly on your voice, Karl – I just want to make music with you, and see what happens…'

He seemed relieved at this. He'd been quite tense the first time we met, asking me a lot of questions through his computer about what I wanted from him. I suspect that he was sick of people testing him and of trying himself to do things he could not manage. But of course the major problem from the beginning of our work together was just this – trying to find ways for him to play an instrument despite his physical difficulties. Karl's movements at this stage were all *very* small and very controlled. When a normally functioning person intends, for example, to move an arm downwards then the almost subconscious mental 'command' is followed by a rapid response, with the arm-weight 'taking' the arm down as a complete single action. Karl, however, had to think every inch of the movement, and there was no natural force or weight in it – nothing 'bounced'. This meant that when Karl held a drumstick in his hand the slow-motion movement of the stick had a strangely controlled quality to it, and when it finally hit the drum it stopped dead on the surface, hardly making a sound.

We were not, at first, very successful in finding a way of working, but I told Karl clearly that it was as much *my* problem in not being able to get the practicalities right as any failure on his part. The first breakthrough was when he played a tambourine with a heavy wooden beater which fell on the instrument and produced at least some sort of satisfying sound. Following this practical breakthrough also came a musical one. I held the tambourine for Karl and sang on each of his beats. After doing this for a short while he suddenly stopped mid-phrase and I held the note. Karl realised at this moment that *he* was directing the action – that there was a link between his beater and my voice. He looked up and laughed!

Listening back later to the tape of this session, I heard that laugh again and realised that this strange, strangulated inhalation was indeed a vocal production. I wondered if there was any possibility of Karl using this in another way. He gave me the answer in the very next session as we did the same activity – Karl playing the tambourine, me singing to each beat he made. Then, quite spontaneously, he started to sing with me – making the only sound he could, which I had heard earlier as a laugh. There was, however, a definite connection between the vocal sound and the motor action of his arm. Karl was singing to accompany his playing, and at this stage it seemed that he could only use his voice when moving – that somehow the motor action 'allowed' the voice. I also had the feeling that it was largely unintentional and that he felt the significance only after it had happened.

As limited as it was, using his voice opened up another channel that was even more immediate for him than playing. We gradually developed an increasingly flexible and creative way of making music together – with our voices, the tambourine, sometimes supported by the more dramatic possibilities of the piano. At first it tended to be in a simple dialogue form, a call and response. Karl's response, however slow and effortful, was nevertheless intentional and meaningful within the musical context. The form of playing gradually expanded – varying between playing and singing together and in alternation, as a call and response.

For variety, we also found that a gong played with a hard beater gave a satisfying sound, indeed the largest noise Karl could produce on his own. It also encouraged larger arm movements. With the music that I happened to accompany this playing with on the piano, I discovered at this stage how much he enjoyed contrasting styles of music. He was equally at home with an atonal idiom as a sentimental one, and I felt it important to give him access to these different ways of feeling through music. It was perhaps the emotional equivalent of the practical problems of playing – that is, getting as wide a range of experience as possible within extreme limitations. This music, however, was certainly not played at Karl. Now that he knew he was in the musical driving seat, his chief pleasure was in testing whether I was really with him, really following – by suddenly stopping playing in mid-phrase and waiting for my reaction! [◎8]

Karl's playing was still in a sense incredibly limited – a simple pulsed beat in a single tempo. But *he* was in control of how he used his only musical gesture, and my job was to place it in different contexts – rhythmic, melodic and harmonic. His single beats might be, for example, every beat of a simple 4/4 phrase, or the first beat of every bar in a 3/4 melody, and so on. In this way he got not only a stronger feeling of his own intention but also an evolving awareness of how music worked and how we could share intention in it. I had, though, to be careful to stay aware of Karl's breathing rhythm. If I played faster or slower than this he was simply unable to respond and would stop playing. I always felt in him a sense of immense energy and power desperately trying to break free of its constraints, and I could well imagine his sense of frustration. But what he *had* found in making music together with someone was a means of direct communication, human and immediate, in contrast to the only other medium he had available, the mechanical and mediate nature of the computer.

Karl did, however, use his computer to tell his parents that music therapy was the most enjoyable therapy he'd had. They themselves thought that after ten sessions or so he seemed more emotionally stable than for a long time. Another interesting if sad piece of information his parents gave me was that Karl would often speak quite normally when asleep. This was a further indication that his problem with speech was one of linking his intention to the physical mechanisms, not just of damage to the voice.

Karl sang for the whole of the fifth session, and I noticed he was making small melodic shapes, as a kind of enlargement of the single tones he sang. I echoed this back to him and 'amplified' the gesture – making slides between notes and trying to use this to give form to our sung dialogue. As a result there was more flow and connection both in the music and in Karl's flow of motor activity. He was able to direct the music with more precision and awareness, and there was a gradual expansion in the tempo range he could tolerate. I still challenged him, however, by altering the musical context of his playing-singing by unexpected phrasing and changes of tempo – but I always gave *him* the responsibility for continuing the music. At the same time, however, it was as much the music itself which gave him the impulse to move; the qualities of the melody which seemed to give him a coherence and continuity of motor action.

Karl found next that he could sing without playing, and thus he had a further musical choice in his small repertoire – sing or not sing. He also discovered a kind of musical yawn which enlarged his vocal range, and we embarked upon a series of strange-sounding vocal dialogues of tonal swoops and yawns. The music needed to be flexible in tempo and phrasing but with a melismatic character which invited him to sing. Karl was finding his voice, physically and musically.[◎9]

Occasional events would take me aback in showing his problems outside of the little oasis of spontaneity we had found in the music. An example of this came at the end of a session when Karl obviously wanted to hug me. But the sad fact was that what, to most people, is a spontaneous emotional gesture was to him a feat of concentration. His arms gradually raised themselves in slow motion like a robot, but he got there! It was Christmas and he asked me to compose him a carol. I said I would if he provided me with a text, so he went away and produced the most bizarre set of words on his computer. I set it to music and we played it together.

This was one of the ways in which Karl showed increasing initiative, expanding his own possibilities of playing and creativity. In the last three or four sessions he chose the triangle to play and set about finding novel ways of playing it. A labour-saving device he hit upon was to swivel the triangle around (it was hanging from a stand), then let it swivel back while he held the metal beater against it.

Music and the creative musical communication which is possible for Karl in music therapy are now one of his chief needs outside his everyday care. He is now able to do some office-work for his father's business and can be slightly more active in the way he leads his life. But in reality he is still painfully limited in his social and emotional expression and communication. For a man who is still only twenty-seven his life on all levels must feel painfully constraining.

In this light, music for Karl is a compensation in the best sense, giving him back something (however modest) of what his illness has taken away. His computer did not invite him to communicate – the music did. The challenge was to find a way for him to communicate without words but with his voice. Music gave just this, but also the *will* to communicate and a real physical form of sound to that communication – one that created sense which involved not just his movements, but his intentions and feelings in dialogue with another person.

LISTENING GUIDE

[ѡ8] Karl sits on a stool with a cymbal on a stand to the left of his body. With a hard wooden beater in his right hand, he slowly brings his arm up, flicks his wrist at the top and leads the arm diagonally across his body to hit the cymbal. On the piano the therapist's music emphasises both strong up- and down-beats supporting and emphasising the movements of Karl's arm and beater. When Karl's arm is up and ready, each time he glances towards the therapist in the split second before it falls to play the cymbal – sometimes with his half-smile of enjoyment in the togetherness of the playing.

[ѡ9] Karl sits in front of a side-drum, and the taps you can hear at the beginning of the excerpt are made by Karl on the rim of the drum. The therapist sings as he plays the drum, and then Karl also begins to sing – coming into the tonality of the music and leading into a dialogue between the two voices.

CHAPTER 10

Quickening

> I was quickened into motion, my own perceptual and kinetic melody quickened into life by the inner life of music. And in that moment, when the body became action, the leg, the flesh became quick and alive, the flesh became music, incarnate solid music. All of me, body and soul, became music in that moment. (Oliver Sacks)

Karl experienced more dramatically than most of us the essential relationship between music and movement, motion and emotion: those of us, that is, who often sit in classical concerts inhibiting the natural responses of our hands and feet to the music, forced to listen only with our ears. But, as Nietzche remarked, we also listen with our muscles, moving with the music and being moved by it. This chapter investigates how this is a central theme for music therapy.

MUSIC: THE 'QUICKENING ART'

To Karl the fact that music induced a different quality of movement for him was central to how music therapy could be of benefit. But this is not restricted to Karl's case, or just to people with neurological damage. Much of the effectiveness of any music therapy stems from the fact that music *moves* us – physically and emotionally; that it involves us and gives a sense of liveliness. Kant called music 'The Quickening Art' and Oliver Sacks used this rather old-fashioned word 'quickening' to describe his own unusual experience of music which he wrote about in his book *A Leg to Stand On* (1986). Quickening means 'to give life to', 'to impart energy', and I use it in this chapter in the same sense as Sacks, to suggest the way in which music works therapeutically not by giving a mechanical stimulus but by somehow lending some of its qualities of liveliness and motivation to both body and spirit.

MUSIC AS AROUSAL

People often comment that music therapy must be calming – an idea presumedly coming from the received wisdom that music can 'soothe the savage breast'. Yet this is curiously against both much of people's experience and the objective evidence available. Playing or listening to music is, on the contrary, more likely to *arouse* us than send us to sleep.

Experimental studies have steadily accrued investigating the influence of sound (and sometimes only by implication music) on our physiology and mental states.[1] This is often seen as one way of proving the efficacy of music therapy – as the dispenser of these positive benefits. It is also a way of fitting music therapy into the 'medical model' and its theories of treatment. We are, however, on dangerous ground here, since there will always remain an ontological gap between the two phenomena: music and physiology. In the same way as music cannot be explained by its acoustical properties alone, so too its influence on people is more than just its ability to induce physiological effects. There are in fact many diverse stimuli which cause much the same physiological patterns of arousal or relaxation as music does. What is important about music is how it affects us in ways beyond any simple physiological or psychological effect. To take an example from ethnomusicology, John Blacking argued against the idea that drumming is the 'cause' of trance (by way of direct physiological influence) in some African music, in a way which is separated from the whole ritual context (Blacking 1987).

Similarly, whilst any account of the effect of music in the context of music therapy must not ignore the physiological effect of sound, it must concentrate first and foremost on the fact of music as something more than this – as a locus of meaning and feeling within and between people.[2] To move us physically it must also move us emotionally. The experiment made on Herbert von Karajan which was described earlier is a good illustration of this. He showed more physiological arousal conducting a slow (but emotional) passage of music than in the certainly more dangerous procedure of landing his jet. In *Music and the Mind* Anthony Storr perhaps comes closer to the truth of these matters with his modest claim that, 'Rhythm, melody

---

1 These have investigated the influence of sound and music on such diverse areas as respiration, galvanic skin response, gastric motility, pupillary reflex and general motoric activity (see Ruud 1980).

2 This is not to deny or devalue some of the more predictable and mechanical effects of sound on the body, some of which have been used to therapeutic benefit. Both 'ultrasound' and 'vibroacoustic therapy' use mechanically administered sound to make changes in the body structure – the former for surgical purposes, the latter to help with chronic musculo-skeletal disorders (see Wigram *et al.* 1989).

and harmony are all ways of ordering tones so that they interact and form relationships. These ordered sounds resonate with physical processes in ways that we do not fully understand' (Storr 1992).

KINETIC MELODIES

These very phenomena can carry not just a musical but also a therapeutic significance in some circumstances.'There came to my aid now melody, rhythm and music' wrote Oliver Sacks (1986) in his account of his accident in Norway (for the background to this see Chapter 1). As a result of nerve injury Sacks describes how he lost the sense of his own leg as a living thing which moved with the flow of his body as a whole. Instead every movement needed to be thought out, intentionally and artificially. The vital change came unexpectedly when he began to imagine a performance of Mendelssohn's Violin Concerto:

> Suddenly, into the silence, the silent twittering of motionless frozen images – came music... And without thinking, without intending whatever, I had found myself walking easily, *with* the music... In the moment that this inner music started the Mendelssohn, which had been summoned and hallucinated by my soul, and in the very moment that my 'motor music', my kinetic melody, my walking came back – in the self-same moment the leg came back. (Sacks 1986)

Note that this is nothing to do with acoustic sound: the performance happened silently inside Oliver Sacks' head. What is *does* concern is the phenomenon of music as a whole: where music is sound organised to convey some significance; with its elements of melody and rhythm conveying a sense of order and movement.

'To hear music is to hear motion' wrote Zuckerkandl (1973). Conversely there are forms of motion – especially in people and animals – which can be seen to have musical qualities. Whilst a machine merely repeats an action an animate body has a *quality of movement:* flow, continuity, coordination, purpose and direction. An earlier chapter outlined how there could be said to be a 'music of the body' and how a sympathy between this and the music we hear or play could account both for the depth of our relationship to music and how it can be so effective as a therapeutic tool. There seems to be a basic similarity between how both music and the body organise themselves as moving forms in time. Moreover, when illness or handicap interferes with the body's processes music seems to be able to lend it some of its own qualities of organisation and movement.

The organisation of pulse comes first in both music and the body. Rhythm functions to order any succession of events in time and, in health, the complex of rhythmic systems in the body must flexibly entrain with each other. The most mechanical aspects of functioning such as heart beat, breathing and digestion also have the most basic rhythmic characteristics, our principal requirement of them being simply that they continue the same action (though they must retain more flexibility than a machine in order to react to metabolic changes). In illness there is often a disruption of the rhythm, or the coordination of the different rhythms. This is true right up to the most complex functions, including the cerebral rhythms of the brain, and Oliver Sacks has written that music is a 'neurological necessity' to patients whose illness disrupts these, 'When a person has a neurological disease, there is a part of his continuous rhythm which is missing. The music helps revive that missing continuity' (Sacks 1993). Whether walking or talking, most of our willed actions also rely on a rhythmic continuity, and it is immediately perceptible when a person's speech rhythm or step is disrupted. Neuromotor conditions such as Parkinson's disease, neurological damage, cerebral palsy and stroke often involve a loss of the ability to move – either at all, or with any quality of flow, spontaneity or identification with the body. Karl, in the last case study, only found these qualities in his movement when he was 'inside' music, reacting to its 'directions' and his own musical intentions.

Undoubtedly the rhythmic aspect of music gave Karl back some of the 'quickness' and order of his motor action. But perhaps as important as this was melody. Oliver Sacks also talks of recovering the 'kinetic melody' of his movement, using here a term of A.R. Luria, the Russian neurologist who studied what gives direction, flow and naturalness to our motor movements. Whilst rhythm ensures the basic continuity of an action (be this a beat on a drum or the next pace of a leg walking) it provides no intrinsic direction. Melody, however, is the musical solution that helped to maintain in sound the continuity and direction of Karl's movements. Embedded in melody they partake in a musical intention which is a higher-level organisation than that of rhythm alone.

'A succession of tones is a melody when the tones exhibit definite dynamic qualities and, in their succession, reveal a dynamic order', writes Zuckerkandl (1959). These 'dynamic' qualities are not anything to do with acoustical properties, but everything to do with purely musical ones: that is, what sense the music makes to us in terms of its tensions and resolutions and where we feel it to be leading. What, in short, makes us want to complete the last note of a melody or to move or make some gesture to express the shape of a melody that is running in our imagination, 'Hearing tones I move with them; I experience their motion as my own motion. To hear tones in motion is to move together with them' (Zuckerkandl 1959). Melody gives direction to succession and, more than rhythm, seems to embody movement – even though nothing in melody physically moves. Rather than a tone moving through space like a ball, melody is really one tone continually making a relationship to another tone, handing on its impulse like a relay-runner to the next man. Though melody is, empirically speaking, a succession of separate tones in *time*, not in space, its subjective musical effect is to create a sense of musical space – of directions, resolutions and phrased shapes.

Phrasing is a final basic musical component of relevance here. In phrasing rhythm meets melody in the medium-term level of organisation in music where the parts of a melody are joined together so they make musical sense. It is perhaps significant that phrasing is often talked about in terms of breathing, even in purely instrumental music. Musicians talk of letting the music 'breathe', meaning that a sense of shape and articulation needs to be found and expressed. Though it may sound too simple to be true, I and other music therapy colleagues often find that clients with chronic lung conditions such as asthma have difficulty phrasing music.[3]

The elements of phrasing in music also apply to normal speech, which is phrased both as a result of the limits of our breath, but also because of how we want to connect our words and expression together to mean something. In fact any complex motor pattern, including walking, could be said to have some phrased aspect, which is one of the qualities which distinguishes it from purely mechanical action. But equally, pathology disturbs phrasing in playing music, or in speech and movement – tending in all three to lead to a loss of natural shape and ease of movement, of ability to convey meaning and expression. In the music therapy situation, however, the aspect of phrasing can, as with rhythm and melody, often be called out in unexpected ways by the overall musical experience and can give back to the client a sense of that which is normally lost or weakened.

---

3 All the points made in this chapter concerning the relationship between musical components and ways of playing music by clients with certain pathological conditions remain at present at the level of anecdotal observations. Considerable research is needed to explore these issues.

FINDING THE RIGHT MUSIC

This kind of explanation of what happens in Creative Music Therapy contains certain dangers: largely that these basic components of music such as rhythm, melody and phrasing will become separated from the significance of the music as a whole. It is then only a short step to a reductionist approach of prescribing music therapy: rhythm for Parkinson's disease, phrasing for asthmatics and so on. On the contrary, I believe exactly the opposite case to be true: that although the musical elements are the 'ingredients' of both what happens in music and consequently in music therapy, it is music as an undivided whole which quickens – which is to say, gives life and fluency and ease back to a person. And this is mediated through the creative and musical relationship that improvisation in Creative Music Therapy can make accessible to clients. The 'solutions' of rhythm, melody and phrasing are essentially by-products of the basic fact of simply making music together.

The key to this chapter is the connection between motion and emotion, which is the real meaning of 'quickening' – not just a mechanical stimulation of movement. A client whose story comes later in the case studies said, after having played a melody on the piano for the first time as part of a piano duet: 'It's possible to *sing* on the piano. I felt that each tone under my fingers was living, not just mechanical.' Similarly, Dr Cecil Todes, who has written about his life with Parkinson's disease and about his experience of Creative Music Therapy, commented 'music moves me – but it has to be the right music' (Todes 1990). And Oliver Sacks said of one of his patients to whom music was a help, 'Only music which moved her *soul* had this power to move her body. She was only moved by music which moved her' (Sacks 1991).

Finding the 'right music' is where the music therapist can be of most help. For some people the right music is the right style, idiom or emotional tone, so that the music is 'moving' and 'catches' them. As we have seen before, improvisation can search out the precise music for a person, so that when we play together a musical meeting is possible. In contrast, pre-recorded music played passively *to* a person cannot adjust to their physical and emotional needs. Equally it can simply fail to connect to anyone – background pop (or background Mozart) in a hospital ward has few of the qualities of active music making, where both the people and the music are involved and engaged.

Another side of finding the right music for somebody is more practical, though none the less important. In Peter Hoffmann's work with Karl, for example, the music had both to meet his physical limitations whilst at the same time create a challenge to these. At first Karl could only manage one painfully slow beat, and any music which was faster or more complex than his movement gave him no chance of responding. But, as the details of this work showed, when the music was truly *his* music, so too was the motion and the emotion of the music his. It quickened not only his action but also his will to act.

One of the most pernicious aspects of handicap or illness is the erosion of the will or of the sense of oneself as still being able to be spontaneous, creative and sometimes joyful. The potency of music as a help in this situation is where we can really use the word 'quicken' with meaning. For quickening is more than just stimulation; it is more than the effect of sound on physiology. Its real gift is the unexplainable power to animate not just the flesh but also the spirit – to give an impulse which makes someone *want* to act, want to respond, want to create.

Oliver Sacks writes about his own moment of musical quickening:

> Suddenly, wonderfully, I was moved by the music. The music seemed passionately, wonderfully, quiveringly alive – and conveyed to me a sweet feeling of life. I felt with the first bars of music a hope and intimation that life would return to my leg – that it would be stirred, and stir with original movement, and recollect or recreate its forgotten motor melody. I felt as if life itself was music, or consubstantial with music; that our living, moving flesh itself was 'solid' music – music made fleshy, substantial, corporeal. (Sacks 1986)

For many of our clients music therapy is often the best way of finding access to this 'life in music', an experience at once purely musical but also irreducibly part of the flow of our bodies, thoughts and feelings: of the inner flow of our lives as a whole.

CHAPTER 11

Herr P.

To say things is so difficult, to sing them so easy!

Within minutes of being brought to the music therapy room in his bed Herr P. asked abruptly, 'What precisely is the relationship of music to the healing system?' I think I probably gave a less than adequate answer to a man who was used to quick answers in his career as a successful industrialist. 'My life was always quick – I've always been impatient' he told me. In contrast he was now a dying man of sixty-seven who had been operated on for a brain tumour.

Though always civil, his manner in the first session was abrupt and defensive. The playing we did was continually interrupted by his comments and questions. When I invited him to play a drum which I put at the side of the bed he said 'play a few bars to me'. He soon joined in, however, and for a man weak and propped up in bed his playing was surprisingly steady, rhythmic and strong. He played along for a few bars and said 'sounds monotonous – not at all the kind of music I want to play'. He stopped playing and started to tell me about some research he had read about concerning the influence of drumming on the body. He did play again in snatches but was never, in this first session, happy with anything he played. 'Play something I know!', he told me. I obliged with some Bach which he beat time to on the drum. Later in the session he surprised me by being quite happy to sing, in a low gravelly voice. But it had a sense of melody and character – though any attempts at improvising tended to gravitate towards something he already knew. A free melody became a Bavarian folk song, which became *Sur le pont d'Avignon* in a clever metamorphosis. But he ended the session

---

Rachel Verney worked with Herr P. at the Gemeinschaftskrankenhaus in Herdecke, Germany.

touchingly by singing Brahms' *Cradle Song*. 'I hope you were not unsatisfied with me' Herr P. added as he left.

My first thought was that he was unlikely to come back again. In some ways music therapy did not seem to suit him at all. Listening back to the tape there was also very little of real musical significance to suggest he had been engaged by the experience. Yet there was a curious blend of contradictory currents in that first session: from the formal to the sentimental; the abrupt to the soft and vulnerable.

I was still unprepared, however, for the difference in the second session just two days later. Herr P. came in and sang a warm and unembarrassed hello to me, then continued singing a monologue (a habit he continued for the rest of the sessions we had together): 'The night can sometimes be better than a beautiful morning...' He sang how he meditated on his life in the night and explained to me (in song) how 'to say things is so difficult, to sing them so easy...'. In comparison to this freedom of expression he continued to be unhappy about the music he improvised on instruments. He wasn't comfortable improvising – in a sense he could not allow himself to improvise freely, to dare to let things happens. He tried to steer the music towards something he knew, or some idiom he was familiar with. The bargain we came to in this session was that I would play some Bach for him to play along with on the drum. This time, however, Herr P. was not just 'shadowing' my playing but playing *with* me, as an additional part. His beat had life and energy as it picked out the sense of dance in the Bach, and the melodic rhythm. But, above all, his playing at last had continuity and engagement. Paradoxically, he *is* the Bach in a way he was never his own music. It was also more of a genuine musical dialogue between us: we brought out qualities in both the Bach and in each other's playing. In one way this was an end in itself: he loved the Bach, it gave him an active and creative contact with the music that had always enriched his life. But from the point of the music therapy it was also a half-way house in that it gave him the confidence to improvise more freely in the final sessions.

I told him at the end of the second session that it was unlikely we could meet the next week as I would probably be at a conference in America. He sung his answer to me, a monologue about the nature of choices: 'In twenty years time you will question your decision to go to America, whether it was right to go or to stay here and give Herr P. a session!'

I did go to the conference and the next session I had with Herr P. was ten days after the last. He sung to me almost straight away, 'you have no idea how much I *long* for this music'. I was still surprised at the seeming change of heart and how the music had taken hold of him. In this and the next two sessions his playing (mostly on drums whilst I played the piano) became surer, more straightforward and more meaningful, whilst physically he became weaker. We also sang a lot – long monologues and duets. A characteristic of both his playing and singing was its cheerfulness, which at times was genuine, but at others seemed agonisingly forced as he battled against pain. But his preference for major keys and jolly rhythms was also related to his love of Bavarian folk music and of ballroom dancing, which I found out he had done for much of his life.

The contradiction between his physical state and the music he wanted to make was most glaringly obvious in the sixth session when he came in chronic pain and lasted just eight minutes. Despite this he wanted to play bumptious, Bavarian-style music. 'I want to live my life happily – you've got to be a *fröhliches Mädchen* for me' he said.

In the next session his pain was under control, and the happiness in the music was natural rather than forced. He sang hello to me in the style of a Bavarian waltz: 'Let's sing a jolly song.' His playing was now controlled and more simple and direct. He would initiate changes in the speed and the style of the music. The main improvisation in this session was a romping, energetic, ballroom-style dance music which he played on two drums, one either side of the bed (he was now too weak to sit up in bed, but for this short time seemed to galvanise extraordinary energy). We were now really making music together, it was fully our own music and it had such vibrancy and vitality – qualities now quite unavailable to him in the world outside music [Ʊ10]. As I saw his life shrinking the intensity and vitality of his music grew – there was no doubt about this. We sang together at the end of the session, and Herr P. sang of his anxiety at going home in the next few days.

The last and eighth session was just before he went home. He was weak and lying down in the bed, but played a first improvisation of ferocious drumming on two drums. He was listening acutely though, and the strong dissonant music eventually calmed down into a quiet passage where there was particularly close musical dialogue between us.

'Let's play Bach' he said, and played his own part on the drum with a sensitivity and character as never before. It had a sprung, dancing rhythm as he beat the melodic rhythm of the music. It had life, vitality and commitment [Ʊ11]. 'I must have some of this at home as well' Herr P. commented. I found out later that he had indeed made his wife go out and buy a drum and cymbal. She was a pianist, but until then they had never been able to make music together. When he came home from the hospital, however, they played together for the remaining three months of his life.

At the end of the last session we sang together as usual, and Herr P. gradually led the music around to a major key, the happy resolution he looked for. He began a sung dialogue between us with:

> 'Auf Wiedersehen...'
>
> 'We'll meet again in this world or the next...'
>
> 'I have already ordered that...'
>
> 'I'm sure we'll recognise each other...'
>
> 'Yes, I'll be the one in the black patent leather shoes.'

LISTENING GUIDE

[🎧10] Herr P. lies in bed, in pain and too weak to sit up. A large drum and a cymbal stand beside the bed. The therapist on the piano and Herr P. on the drum improvise in the style of a ballroom tango. They play together with the energy and flair of dancing partners. The music is mainly fast, often syncopated. Herr P. plays the dance with a surprising stability and strength, animated with enthusiasm and enjoyment.

[🎧11] Herr P. says 'Let's play Bach' and the therapist plays the Prelude no.5 in F. Herr P. plays along with this on the drum, and although too weak to control his playing all the way through, he is extremely sensitive to the style and the melodic rhythyms, at times playing with strength, precision and decisiveness. The quality of his playing is again lively and dance-like.

CHAPTER 12

David

The invention of melody is the supreme mystery of Man. (Claude Lévi-Strauss)

'I bet you don't know what that was?', David asked me, suddenly stopping playing the drum. 'Well, it sounded like quite a complicated rhythm', I answered. 'I'll tell you' he continued, 'this is the Piccadilly line before it gets into Leicester Square [demonstrates], and *this* after [further demonstration].'

In the first session with David the rhythm of the Piccadilly line kept cropping up: part show-off, part joke and part test of me. It seemed an almost autistic gesture, yet David was not autistic. But this was only one of a long list of paradoxes that uncovered themselves in the three years we worked together. David was a man in his mid-thirties who was often child-like in his naivety and vulnerability, yet also a born performer. He was a man who calculated the mathematical ratios of sound frequencies, but also once answered, when I asked him if he felt sad, 'what's "sad"?'

David was born blind and his handicap reinforced by a childhood which not only failed to help him, but further damaged him, emotionally and socially. Though he had no formal psychiatric condition there were chronic and deep-seated emotional problems which the little help he had been given so far had not managed to deal with. Indeed much of his life was a tragic story of failing to get the help he needed at the right time, and of being abandoned by the people who could have helped. An emotionally disturbed childhood had meant that he had fallen into the cracks of the then rudimentary education for the blind, failed to learn Braille or cope in any but the most basic way with his handicap. He now worked a forty-hour week in a factory assembling costume jewellery, where only one person could speak English with him. Just from the evidence of our work in music alone this was clearly a tragic waste.

Not that David was an easy person to help. At different times efforts had been made and had failed, largely due to the paranoid side to his personality which could quickly turn on people and could be frightening. It was less intentional aggression than a response like that of a frightened animal. This may not be too far from the truth of how David saw himself, as he would talk of his 'claws' and 'paws', or his 'gills'. To him there were two groups of people: a few friends he could trust, the rest 'enemy' as he would say, ready to harm him. This gross distortion in his emotional perception often meant that he simply misinterpreted innocent attempts at help, and regularly got into fights on the tube when some well meaning person had simply given him a helping hand on the escalator. Yet David still wanted to make contact with people, but he simply did not know how. 'They told me I'm not good at relating with people', he said once, 'they' presumably being some agency who had assessed David without finding a way to help him. He was referred to music therapy from a counselling service where attempts at help had been less than successful. David had mentioned music and it was thought that this might just be a way in.

My first questions were how, in the jargon, David's 'primary handicap' (his blindness) related to the 'secondary handicap' (his emotional and communication problems). A book came out while I was working with David which gave me a clearer insight into his world: John Hull's record of his own blindness, *Touching the Rock* (1991). The following passage I found especially helpful:

> It makes me realise the inflexibility of the blind, or I should say the inflexible kind of life imposed on people by blindness. Familiarity, predictability, the same objects, the same people, the same routes, the same movement of the hand to locate this or that: take these away, and the blind person is transported back into the infantile state where one simply does not know how to handle the world, how to enter into it and control it, how to exist in a relationship to that world, where the hard-won balance between trust and fear threatens to be upset, and one is overwhelmed by the thought that the world to which one seeks to be related is unrelateable to, because either it is unreal or unavailable. It is inhabited by beings to whom it does belong, the sighted. The world which then remains is one's body, the introspective consciousness. This is a world into which the sighted cannot penetrate, a place where some kind of inner control can be established. This is to go back beyond infancy into the unborn state, where one is free-floating without distinction, enclosed at the the end of the tunnel, without a world and, finally, without a self. (Hull 1991)

Many of these qualities – the inflexibility, the tug between trust and fear, the tight boundary between self and world, could be heard directly in David's playing. At first he chose non-melodic instruments and played in a dominating way, with obsessively controlled rhythms built up like a defensive wall of sound. It felt like a show of musical force, I felt pulled and pushed along by it as I tried to play with him on the piano. We both played but it felt like a monologue I was supporting, not that we were playing together. [☋12]

It was much the same on any of the instruments he tried, percussive or melodic. The xylophone, for example, was played with the same fast, obsessive rhythms as the drum. [☋13] Though all the playing had a driven quality, none of it had continuity or natural flow, and would simply come to a halt when he got stuck. He was then dependent on me to provide a new idea. The result was a confusing blend of musical hostility combined with dependence, perhaps the result of the simple fact that he did not trust me. I wrote in my notes after the first session:

> There's something child-like about David: demanding attention for his desire to perform and dominate. Hard to tell the level of anxiety beneath the bravado. His social awkwardness parallels in the music; where obvious close musical listening (demonstrated by speed of response at cadences, etc.) is coupled by insensitivity to allowing me a word in edgeways! Desire to impress me, be clever-clever in picking out tunes, etc. Felt *some* degree of musical rapport. Can hear more evidence of dialogue on the tape than I heard in the session (his playing felt very over-bearing).

Nevertheless David turned up every week and really worked at the situation for a full three years. This was new to him – to find something which both helped him and yet centred on something he found he *could* do and could enjoy, where he felt comfortable and appreciated. And the fact was that he had real talent for music, talent that like most of his potential had been undetected, let alone nurtured. Though there were factors which seemed at first to obscure his musical sensitivity I could feel it was there. Though David had never had a music lesson he had spent much of his life listening to music on the radio; listening I suspect with more care than many of us, assimilating the 'rules' of music passively. His work in music therapy was in one sense a committed practical exploration, even perhaps you might say an experiment in music. One by one he seemed to discover the 'workings' of music and of musical communication – but in his own terms, without theory. Often these purely musical discoveries seemed also to be a pilot for a change in his emotional and social life.

Establishing trust between us took a full six months. This was not just David's need to test the fact that I would not, like most before, give up and leave him after a while. It was also the discovery of a musical trust which laid the foundation of our dialogue. At the beginning David played and I played 'beside' him; echoing, accompanying, supporting. But I rarely felt he was really letting me play *with* him, that there was any space left for us to meet musically. If we chanced to meet too closely in the music David would subvert this with some odd verbal comment like 'bet you can't play a tune that doesn't exist!', which succeeded in breaking the mood.

But the fact was that David was listening from the beginning, was acutely aware of the sense of the music, and after a while could not but begin to share some of this sense between us. He discovered musical dialogue in improvisation, beginning with the simplest devices such as turn-taking with question and answer phrases, exchanging of motifs and rhythms, cadencing together.

The first session David had come and promptly set up his cassette recorder and microphone in the corner. I was quite taken aback by this since, though I tape sessions myself, I usually try to dissuade a client from listening back to the sessions themselves when they occasionally ask if this would be possible.[1] I did not, however, want to upset David at the time, and he continued to tape every session. I knew that he listened back to the session several times during the week at home and I often thought about *how* David listened to these tapes. Obviously it would not have been in the same way as me, with my conscious 'theory' of music therapy. In one sense David listened to it purely as music and told me 'that was good music, last week!'. Yet this is to underestimate the subtlety that he developed in his listening. Again the comments that he made occasionally showed that he was aware of hearing rapport, creativity and *how* other people were listening within the music (when he later played in a music therapy group). 'There was a lot of listening going on in that group, last time' was a typical comment he would make. In this light we were both listening to the tapes of the sessions in the same way: namely, that the quality of the relationship in the music and the quality of listening determined both how well the music 'worked' and how satisfactory the experience felt to the players.

Musical dialogue may have been at first a rather stilted form of turn-taking, but it was at the same time a vital transition to *sharing* our musical worlds.

1 There are several reasons for this. The client may be discouraged if it seems to sound a mess to them, or possibly be encouraged to repeat the good bits in the next session. I do, however, often compile a tape of 'highlights' for a client at the end of working with them.

It gradually became more natural and fluid and David became increasingly aware of how an open dialogue releases creativity, how we could find musical meaning together even though an improvisation was not something he could control. He said himself:

> I found after a while I could really make my own music...we knew what to do together...I mean, it's making a musical conversation together really – I'm talking to you through the xylophone, you're talking to me through the piano. It's like that last piece – that I composed in just the *one* go...I listened to your chords and the way you played them, then I worked out the notes on here [xylophone] roughly with your notes, that's how I tried to do it. How can I make something out of it? I don't know if I even think that...I said to that lady the other day, you just come out with a noise and then out of that noise comes something recognisable...and out of that noise came that tune...which I did myself![2]

There was a very gradual but real change in David's musical world which was surprisingly closely paralleled in how he changed in general. Hostility and defensive playing led to more listening and shared dialogue; obsessively 'closed' rhythm and melody led to more flexibility and musical space; safe predictability by invention and creative experiment. John Holt, in the passage quoted earlier, wrote of the 'hard-won battle between trust and fear'. David seemed to have had come to a distorted and damaging compromise on this spectrum when I first met him, but there were signs that musically, emotionally and socially he was moving towards a state of more trust and less fear.

Yet I was nervous about our sessions being the only positive thing in his life, which was otherwise limited and isolated. He was comfortable with me and the narrow confine of the music therapy situation, but what of the fear and distrust he still held for all but the few 'good' people (in his terms)? I also ran a music therapy group at this time (see Chapter 19), part of whose purpose was to provide something for people like David. Yet I was nervous to introduce him too soon, since he could seldom cope with people he did not know, let alone in a group. If I am honest I also have to add that I was afraid David would upset the group, given his very occasional panic-induced outbursts could be quite disturbing.

---

2 David could not fill out the questionnaire I gave to the group and asked me if I could interview him on tape instead. He talked both of the group and of his individual sessions with me and gave me permission to use his comments in any way I needed.

I took courage in the end and David joined the group, where up to ten people met weekly to improvise music together. It was a drop-in group so there were often new members or visitors. David was predictably frightened at first and barricaded himself in the corner with a xylophone, not making any contact with anyone else, and to an extent regressed to his old musical persona: play a lot so that nobody else can get in! This time, however, his easing out of this was quicker, but followed the same pattern as had my work with him in the individual sessions. He heard himself being heard, being answered *within* the music and began to make contact with people purely musically at first. He explains it himself:

> The music helped me like the people...when I first joined it took me a long time to even speak to people. With 'x' we were playing the xylophones together. She said afterwards 'I liked what you did' and I said 'I liked what you did too'...and we became friends!

It happened that, quite independently, as part of the questionnaire I gave to the group to help me with a report, 'x' also writes of just this event from her side:

> I soon found that I could have a dialogue musically with David that was richer and more interesting than any spoken conversation we'd had. At first we would listen to each other and echo what we heard. As we grew more confident, we could respond with variations on the theme – then, later, adding interesting rhythmic variations and counterpoint. I think we both enjoyed it and it helped form our friendship. David is a man who otherwise I don't believe I ever could have got to know, or to like and accept. The music therapy forged the relationship.

David made other relationships this way, sometimes answering people musically in the other corner of the room. He found himself appreciated and liked, and gradually managed to tolerate the anxiety which he felt every time there was somebody he did not know in the group. I knew something important was changing when one day, after he had played in a musical dialogue with a visitor to the group, he went to find that person after the improvisation in order to talk to her and tell her that she'd played well.

A particular musical friend he made in the group was a woman who came only infrequently. As two people they seemed especially incompatible, yet as two musical 'voices' it worked perfectly. She would sometimes bring her flute and David eagerly asked one day if they could play a duet together. His newly found speciality was a rather nasty plastic instrument called a melodica, which is a cross between a recorder and a mouth-organ (though it has a full chromatic keyboard). It is usually quite useless for music therapy purposes and lay hidden in the cupboard. David discovered it and learned to play it, transforming its basic raucousness into a beautiful tone. In one of the groups the flute and the melodica stood side by side and improvised a duet, accompanied gently by the other players in the room. The improvisation quickly found its focus and weaved a two-part counterpoint with the two voices. To call this two-part counterpoint, however, is to conjure up something intellectual, which was far from the intuitive way they found of combining their two musical voices through a degree of listening, equality and invention. To many of the rest of us it was a jolt against the way we had previously seen these two people. [ʊ14]

As with every case study the positive aspects get emphasised at the expense of the crises and frustrations. Every so often there would be some incident which would re-awaken all David's old patterns, when fear once again would eat at the trust gained. For three months, starting from a trivial misunderstanding, David refused to speak to anyone but me at the practice where we worked. He particularly upset the receptionist, who was one of the people he had dared to get to know in the last year. Recovery after each crisis, however, seemed quicker and David stuck it out instead of running, his previous response to any form of trouble. I came into the reception area after the solution to this incident to find David and the receptionist sitting together accompanied by his gesture of reconciliation, the gaudiest bunch of flowers I have ever seen. David evidently had the idea that more colours means better, and had instructed a puzzled florist to make a bunch of every different flower in the shop!

The two music therapy situations, individual and group, complemented each other, and developments – musical and personal – fed each other. In three years of session both David and I have literally hundreds of tapes of our music. It is in a way daunting to trace the complex development of his playing, and I am genuinely shocked at the difference between the later playing (which I have in my mind as 'characteristic') and the qualities of the playing in the first year. Yet one simple, perhaps simplistic, phenomenon stands out from all the complexity: the discovery of melody. Claude Lévi-Strauss, in the sentence quoted as the epigraph to this case study, describes melody as an invention, 'the supreme mystery of Man'. Of course, David heard melody and to an extent played melodically on the xylophone from the beginning. But it was melody dominated by rhythm, not melody whose motion came from inner direction rather than outer compulsion. David's intuitive discovery of 'real' melody came gradually but surely: it became less 'tight', rhythmically driven and four-square and more fluid, exploratory; it had more space. As I watched David walking across the room one day to fetch an instrument the penny dropped. David *had* no 'real' space as we, the sighted, have. His 'space' was measured time – the distance across the room was ten unconsciously measured paces. His way of walking gave it away; a downward plod without real direction. David had no vista, nothing to see *towards*; there was no space in his world, since it contracted into time, or into the private, bounded space of his own body. This seemed to make perfect sense in terms of the way he played music. At first the 'space' of melody became contracted into the 'time' of rhythm. David's 'discovery' of melody in music was also, I think, a discovery of a sense of space in himself which extended literally out into the world.

The perfect example of this new sense of melody came when David found another instrument hidden in the cupboard, a cheap electronic keyboard that I had never found a use for. It made generally unpleasant sounds, but between us we found just one bearable option, a synthesised flute. David went on to produce an improvisation of pure melody in the truest sense: a Fauré-esque ark of perfectly balanced phrases, rising and falling in dialogue with my simple chordal accompaniment. It has the feeling of all great melody: that it knows exactly where it is going, and could not be otherwise. Yet it was improvised, a fact several audiences in music colleges who I have played this extract to in talks have refused to believe. [♫15]

This quality of melody not only gave a sense of direction to his own musical experience, it gave us a *shared direction* in our playing together, with the melodic and harmonic elements influencing each other. We were not just synchronised in the same beat, but had an experience of thinking, of feeling the life of the melody together – a sharing not just of the present but of the future. Above all, though, in this and other improvisations we shared the sheer beauty that happened between us in music, a level I am convinced that he seldom experienced in other parts of his life.

This musical experiment continued with more subtle exploration of melodic and harmonic areas. This was never a conscious attempt to learn something like a music student: it arose instead from an intuitive need on David's part to expand his musical expression. Whilst I was uncompromising in never letting him stick in a cosy pattern, he was equally unremitting in his will to keep pushing against the walls of his musical self. In a purely empirical way he successively 'discovered' musical dialogue, motivic construction, extended melody, rhythmic and melodic counterpoint, chromaticism, diminution and augmentation, rudimentary harmony...David knew none of these terms and was quite unable to understand them conceptually. But perhaps more than anyone I have ever played music with, he understood them as real musical phenomena: which exist solely within the purely musical law and exist solely with the purpose of laying the ground of musical creation and communication. This he understood perfectly.

I asked David at the end of our time together whether the sessions had helped. 'It helped me bring up my knowledge of music...even to mix with people.' As a music therapist I might be tempted to reverse this: to put the changes in his emotional and social experience and behaviour above what he gained in musical experience. But with David 'musical knowledge' was not something separated from him: it was rather a journey within the depths of the phenomenon of music and of his own creativity. This in itself led naturally to a new quality of experience with other people. Who am I to say which is the more important?

David was pleased when a new radio station called 'Classic FM' was launched in London and which broadcasted accessible and varied classical music. For the last few months of our sessions David came with his head full of good tunes, from Debussy to Purcell, each cleverly adapted to the melodica. They expanded our repertoire of idioms, and David was happy to improvise out of the tunes. He played Purcell's *Trumpet Tune* so well that I suggested he performed it with me accompanying at the forthcoming Christmas concert. David agreed and, frightened as he was, performed with a sense of dignity and musical commitment that created one of those moments when an audience really is caught. David said later, 'People clapped and they cheered and I knew that I'd done well!'

LISTENING GUIDE

[12] David plays a side drum with a single beater. As the music gathers speed and force the compulsive quality of his playing at this time can be heard. But it is also clear how carefully David is none the less listening – demonstrated by how controlled a 'ritardando' both players manage towards the end of the excerpt.

[13] David plays a xylophone with one beater – a feat of dexterity to play with such rhythmic exactness these fast melodic patterns. The playing is energetic but has a driven, breathless quality.

[14] David plays the melodica, 'x' flute and the therapist piano, with other members of the group accompanying on various percussion instruments. The excerpt fades in after approximately one minute of the start of the improvisation, with all three main players. After a cadence the piano is left playing alone for a short time, after which the flute and melodica enter one after another. It is important to know here that neither player was 'conducted in' at this point but chose to play. For the remainder of the excerpt melodica, flute, piano and accompanying instruments play together.

[♫15] David plays with his right hand only on an electronic keyboard programmed with a 'flute voice'. The excerpt fades in after a few minutes of the start of the improvisation. It is important to remember that David has no training in playing a keyboard and that he cannot see what he is doing or have any visual contact with the therapist (who plays piano at the other side of the room).

CHAPTER 13

Creating

> To produce is to draw forth, to invent is to find, to shape is to discover. In bodying forth I disclose… The work produced is a thing among things, able to be experienced and described as a sum of qualities. But from time to time it can face the receptive beholder in its whole embodied form. (Martin Buber)

DARING TO CREATE

When I introduced myself as the music therapist Mr W. looked uncomfortable. 'I don't think it's for me', he said, 'I'm a desk man myself: it's my wife who does all the creative side.' Much the same logic is found in our culture as a whole, with creative activity normally left to someone else: the artist, the professional, the gifted few. It is not that we make too little of creativity, but rather too much. As a member of a music therapy group I was involved in said, 'I always thought of myself as totally incapable of being creative, of communicating or contributing musically, and it was a delight to find that I could, and that music was not just the province of the "experts".' There is also the refreshingly pragmatic statement made by David, from the last case study: '*That* I composed in just the *one* go!… You just come out with a noise, and then out of that noise comes something recognisable…and out of that noise came that tune…which I did myself!'

David had none of the usual inhibitions about what his music should sound like, of how talented he needed to be before even daring to create. He simply started. This was perhaps the child-like aspect of him which could bear to do something for its own sake without worrying about the outcome. Another way of putting this would be to say that David felt free to play. It is perhaps no coincidence that we talk of 'playing music', and no trivialisation of music that it has associations with 'playing' in its more everyday sense.

Indeed Thomas Clifton (1983) has gone so far as to call play a 'primary essence' of music, and as such a sometimes forgotten way in which music is importantly different from verbal language. 'Playing on words' is indeed possible, but not a fundamental use of language – whereas music is somehow *always* play (however serious).[1] Some adults coming to Creative Music Therapy for the first time fear that it will be childish, especially when the sight of the percussion instruments reminds them of school music. Often, however, a more fundamental worry is of playing itself (in both senses): of its being something spontaneous, improvised, exploratory and, above all, something done for its own sake with an emphasis on the process rather than the product.

These qualities of play are also the basic ingredients of creativity: in whatever field (scientific or artistic), at whatever level and in whatever medium. The name of the approach presented in this book – Creative Music Therapy – states clearly both its essence and its priority. It is first and foremost about creativity in music and creativity between people *through* music. It takes as a principle that to be musical is to be creative and to be creative is itself therapeutic because it fulfils some of our basic needs: to find new experiences, new patterns, new meanings; to act freely, flexibly and spontaneously. Some of these needs can be satisfied when we create alone, some are reliant on the additional spur of creative dialogue between people.

Writing and defining creativity is, however, a dangerous enterprise, and within a clinical sphere its investigation is known as a researcher's graveyard. This chapter, then, is not an attempt to build yet another theory of creativity, but a more modest investigation of how creativity is central to what happens in Creative Music Therapy. This is less concerned with creativity as an abstract fact, but with the experience of being creative, and of the physical, emotional and social conditions which sometimes interfere with a person's ability to find this state.

CREATIVITY AND THERAPY

One of the possible etymologies for our word 'creativity' is the Greek for 'fulfilling'. This suggests both how, in creative acts, a piece of music or a painting comes into the world as a new form and how this can in turn bring about an inner experience of fulfilment for the creator. This, moreover, is not just an intellectual experience but involves our feelings, bodies and (in music

---

1 'it would be wrong to think that music *represents* play. It has no need to do this since it *is* play even in its most serious manifestations' (Clifton 1983).

particularly) a quality of communication with other people. In contrast to feeling limited, dull and stuck the experience of being creative involves a motivation and an energy (that we sometimes call inspiration).

Theories of creativity abound, both philosophical and psychological. Though this is not the place for a detailed survey of these, one particular set of ideas – from the psychoanalytical tradition – are of relevance to how creativity has often been understood within the art therapies, and how Creative Music Therapy both agrees with and takes issue with some of these ideas.

Taking their cue from Freud's studies of Leonardo and Michelangelo, psychoanalytic writers at first concentrated on the psychological motivations of the great artists, rather than on creativity as a universal phenomenon. Freud seemed in fact to view creativity (or at least the motivation for it) as a symptom of maladjustment.[2] This, however, was one of the areas in which both those who followed him and those who reacted against him have differed. Jung and Melanie Klein both saw the process of creativity in a more positive light than Freud and incorporated creative aspects into their therapeutic approaches. Maslow and Winnicott wrote extensively about creativity as both a normal and an essential process for human psychological health, and something which was not just the province of the experts but available to everyone.

That the development of the arts therapies followed somewhat in the shadow of the psychotherapies had the consequence that psychodynamic ideas about creativity have had an influential effect on their theory and practice. This has led to the tension that, whilst to the artist creativity and the resulting art-works stand simply for their own sakes, it is a characteristic of psychodynamic approaches that creativity (or play) has another motive. Jung's process of 'active imagination',[3] for example, used play and creative processes, but with the conscious intention of gaining access to an inner psychological reality through the transitional medium of the imagination. Likewise, for many arts therapies following the psychodynamic tradition, the art-product is to be consciously used for interpretation and verbal processing.

---

2 Anthony Storr makes an extensive critique of this idea in his book *The Dynamics of Creation* (1976).

3 'The art of letting things happen, action through non-action, letting go of oneself... became for me the key opening the door to the way' Jung, quoted in A. Stevens, *On Jung* (1991).

It would be fair to say, however, that D.W. Winnicott, a psychoanalytic writer who has influenced many creative therapists, is more aware than most of the dangers in this area. Through his work with children he studied the nature of play and later how a 'play model' fitted into his concept of what happens in psychotherapy. He was always careful to emphasise, however, that his ideas were not a psychoanalytic explanation of play but of how play and creativity were relevant to healthy functioning and to its attempted restitution within a psychotherapeutic relationship. 'It is always good to remember' he wrote 'that playing is itself a therapy', 'the basis of what we do is the patient's playing, a creative experience taking up space and time, and intensely real for the patient...this observation helps us to understand how it is that psychotherapy of a deep-going kind may be done without interpretative work' (Winnicott 1991). Winnicott formulated the concept of 'primary creativity' to express the sense in which all of us, beginning at birth, create our world – forging a personal web of inner meanings and outer objects and actions. This view does not limit creativity to self-consciously artistic pursuits but includes spontaneous play, imagination, and what might be called an attitude of 'creative living' in the most general way. In this sense creativity is seen as much as a capacity than an actual process: with any creative act, at any level, being underpinned by a more basic 'emotional creativity'. This denotes the *capacity* in a person for a certain range of qualities: for autonomy which is nevertheless sensitive to outside influence; for flexibility, confidence, imagination; for the ability to tolerate uncertainty. Conversely, it is clear that someone with the opposite qualities is unlikely to have the capacity either to create artistic objects or to live creatively in the world in Winnicott's sense.

Winnicott concluded that psychological illness[4] can be seen as the degree to which creativity, in the above sense, was hidden and that:

> It is creative apperception more than anything else that makes the individual feel that life is worth living. Contrasted with this is a relationship to external reality which is one of compliance, the world and its details being recognised but only as something to be fitted in with or demanding adaptation. (Winnicott 1991)

4 Winnicott writes as a psychoanalyst about psychological illness. Many music therapists work, however, with a range of clients with chronic illness and have come to much the same conclusion as Winnicott.

Winnicott's ideas deal with an area which is the everyday working reality of all arts therapists – the overlap between 'emotional creativity' and 'artistic creativity' or, to put it another way, between the client's personal *capacity* to be creative and how this is part of the actual concrete creative process of playing music, painting or dancing. The therapist's job is to make each work for the other – teasing out the basic capacity to create whilst relying on the impact of those moments of creativity and success in the work to encourage and give confidence.

Because these issues are so fundamental, Winnicott's ideas can also be useful to creative therapists *not* working to a specifically psychodynamic model. At the same time they are no more an adequate explanation of what happens in Creative Music Therapy than any other non-musical model. They do, nevertheless, provide a useful way of understanding how creativity is relevant to individual health and to therapeutic intervention.

DARING TO PLAY

I quoted earlier, in the chapter on improvisation, the client who reported 'sometimes when I was really flowing, the music seemed to play itself through me. These were the most exciting times for me. Perhaps you might say that my inner musician was allowed out fully to PLAY.' Another, about her experience of a music therapy group, commented:

> There was an atmosphere in which I felt free to experiment, and even to 'fail'. There is so little room for attempting and failing – and the space to do that in creative endeavours seems critical to me.'Fail' is a bad word perhaps, but the fact that there was no judgement on the end product – that the focus was on the process was such a relief.

'Playing' and experimenting are closer to a child's experience than the average adult's, who even taking part in amateur music is often more occupied in 'being right' than being creative. For this reason improvisation is a great help in music therapy to encourage creativity, since we start from the understanding that nothing can be 'right' or 'wrong', that we will simply see what happens. Admittedly, when I explain this to someone coming to music therapy for the first time and ask them just to start, I often get a despairing look, or 'I can't – I don't know what!' Yet in 99 per cent of cases when that person has dared to play 'anything' then we are seconds away from an improvisation beginning to find its own shape and impetus. In David's words, 'out of that noise came something recognisable'. Without having prepared anything, without reproducing anything already composed, we can nevertheless build a musical structure through our creative dialogue.

It can start from a single note, rhythm or texture. Improvisation is often called 'free improvisation' because it relies on a chain of free decisions, on simply doing next what seems inevitable, what 'fits' as the music is carried along on the wave of its own logic and the free, creative decisions of the players.

A central theme of this book, that music therapy works in the way music works, requires that we go beyond seeing creativity as a general capacity and towards the examination of specifically *musical* creativity. By this I mean the difference between being creative in making music as opposed to painting or writing. The nuts and bolts of this are, however, difficult to describe non-musically, especially without reference to a specific musical example. Exactly this was attempted, however, in the earlier chapter 'Just a Minute...', to which it might be profitable to think back to (if not turn back to) at this point. The two minutes of music therapy there show in microcosm a process of musical creativity in its simplest form: when something came out of nothing, despite the fact that the client expected, on the contrary, nothing to come of nothing!

CREATIVITY AND MUSICALITY

Martin Buber's statement, used as the epigraph to this chapter, expresses well what seems to be happening in both the 'Just a Minute...' example and in much improvisation in general: that to produce is to draw forth, to invent is to find, to shape is to discover. This is not to suggest a type of what has been called 'musical platonism',[5] where the musical form is already complete and is just somehow incarnated by the composer or improviser. Rather I mean that there is a process of finding and discovering meaningful connections within the potential of the material in relationship to our imagination. Further to this I want to suggest two forms of creative dialogue which are relevant to Creative Music Therapy: the first between the client and the music (as her 'raw material'); the second a creative dialogue between client and therapist *in* the music.

The intra-creative process

The first of these, what we might call the 'intra-creative process'[6] is always a form of play, however serious the intent. Be it a composer or a client in music therapy, he begins with a playful dialogue of discovery within his

5 For a fuller and fascinating treatment of this issue see the chapter 'Musical Platonism' in Kivy (1993).

6 These two terms are borrowed from Mercedes Pavlicevic.

inner, imaginative world and the precise qualities and potentials of his chosen material of sound (which are in the world of objects). This begins with a 'playing around' with the sounds of the instruments, and then of how to combine them and how to combine them meaningfully and imaginatively to make sound that makes sense. The results are not just an abstract pattern but one which relates to that person's immediate bodily experience, as in improvisation he discovers the relationship of the rhythmic and tonal aspects of his body and action to the form and character of the music he creates.[7]

'She's very musical' is a phrase we often hear to describe someone who has not just a technical grasp of an instrument but also some creative and imaginative relationship to the world of music. Musicality, I would tentatively suggest, is what we mean by the specifically musical type of creativity I am concerned with in this section. Musicality, like creativity, seems to denote less a thing in itself but a *quality* of a person's relationship to music. As with creativity, the concept of 'musicality' is often used to describe the gifted few – and indeed it is undeniable that there are aspects of musicality which are the result of particular gifts, training and experience. But, as creativity is not just about masters and masterpieces, neither is musicality just a question of skill or sophistication. A child's singing can be musical; a client in music therapy with no musical training can be musical, whilst there is at least the possibility of a trained musician in the same situation playing in a rigid and uncreative way – musical only in the sense of using his musical knowledge and experience, not in the immediate qualities of his playing.

Whilst the music therapist is certainly not looking to develop the client's skill in playing music as such, she *is* involved in uncovering musicality in the above sense. This is because musicality is related to more general qualities which are very much the concerns of music therapy: of creativity, flexibility, imagination and a sense of the playing coming from the whole person, a balance of thought and feeling. Perhaps, tellingly, it is easier to recognise

---

7 Danah Zohar, in her book *The Quantum Self* (1990) illustrates the 'intra-creative' process nicely with her example of a child making a clay pot: 'The whole process by which the child makes the pot is a chain of free decisions. In making the pot he gives shape and meaning to something which had never existed before. He draws together a hitherto unexpressed idea in himself and a so-far unmoulded collection of clay molecules, and transforms both into a new thing which *is* the relation of his idea to that clay. More than that, it is the relation of himself, of his evolving sense of beauty, to that clay. The child's creative act has given rise to a new thing (the pot), to a new articulation of his sense of beauty, and to an incarnation of the relationship between the child, his sense of beauty and the clay pot. Thus, in making the pot, the child has also made some aspect of himself and some small portion of his world – his relationship to things.'

the qualities of un-musical playing: rigid, mechanical, compulsive, uninventive or inflexible playing which is uninvolved and unspontaneous. These qualities, moreover, will almost certainly relate not just to the music but to the more basic 'emotional creativity' of the player – an area often interfered with by illness or handicap in the clients music therapists work with. Any work in music therapy must consequently involve the realm of musicality in this inclusive sense.

The inter-creative process

Among the arts therapies music therapy is unique in the degree to which the process involves a direct (and usually constant) creative dialogue with the therapist. In contrast to the 'intra-creative process' between client and material, here we can talk of the '*inter*-creative process' which happens *between* the client and therapist. In the earlier chapter 'Meeting', which was devoted to the client–therapist relationship in the music, I used Martin Buber's concept of the 'Between' to talk about a 'musical between': the creative space in which both players improvise the music – which is to do with both of them whilst not being an exclusive personal expression of either. Again, it can be seen from the 'Just a Minute...' example how the two players find form together in the music through their musical response to each other, and in doing so create not just a 'musical object' together but also a quality of relationship between them.

AN UNEQUAL CREATIVITY?

A question which arises for many people concerns what might be called the 'skill discrepancy' between the client and the therapist in the music therapy situation. How, we are asked, can it be in any sense an equal creative relationship when the therapist is a skilled musician, normally playing a piano, whilst the client is mostly (but not always) musically unskilled and playing only a percussion instrument. A first point in answer is that it will I hope be clear from the above that what we work for in Creative Music Therapy is not a level of musical skill but certain *qualities* of creativity and musicality which can be apparent at any level of complexity. Many music therapists work with both children and adults and see it as part of their skill to adjust to whatever musical level is appropriate. What I want to suggest additionally here is that the normal situation in Creative Music Therapy can be a meaningful creative dialogue without needing to be an equal one in every sense. An analogy might help here: that of the players making a musical journey together. Both are travelling through the same musical territory, but one (the conceptually untrained musician – who doesn't have a way of representing music abstractly) is mostly just travelling with the flow, from event to event. She is not, however, just a passive passenger but gives energy, creative ideas and reactions (to a greater or lesser extent) as to where the journey leads. And indeed the feedback from clients suggests that they do not feel they are simply accompanying the therapist's piano-playing but mostly experience themselves being 'in the driving seat'. The difference, however, between the client and the other musical traveller (the therapist – who *is* both practically and 'conceptually' competent) is that he also has a provisional map of the musical territory in his head (from experience and intuition) and an idea of the overall likelihood of the journey. One open to revision, but one there all the same.[8] This by no means indicates (to continue the metaphor) that the client is somehow just being taken for a ride. It does mean, however, that the therapist assures the basic coherence of the musical experience (by virtue of his structurally informed playing) therefore providing the freedom for the more localised creativity and musical intention of the client. Within this situation the therapist can guide and help musically when this is necessary, or leave the creative direction wholly to the client when appropriate. Sometimes considerable help is necessary at the beginning – when someone is simply incapable of making music satisfactorily by themselves.

Another obvious example of a skill discrepancy which nevertheless contains mutual creativity is a verbal or play relationship with a baby or child. Winnicott commented on this and came to a similar formulation of the nature of creative dialogue by looking at play and creativity within the mother–infant relationship:

> It is useful, then, to think of a third area of human living, one neither inside the individual or outside in the world of shared reality. This intermediate living can be thought of as occupying a potential space… The potential space between mother and baby, between child and family, between individual and society or the world, depends on experience which leads to trust. It can be looked upon as sacred to the individual in that it is here that the individual experiences creative living. (Winnicott 1991)

---

8 There is experimental evidence to support this interpretation by music psychologists studying the different strategies of listening to music (see Cook, *Music, Imagination, Culture* 1990).

At best in Creative Music Therapy it is in the 'musical between' (as the musical equivalent of Winnicott's 'potential space') that the client is given not just a musical experience but one of creative living.

A client came recently for individual music therapy after her second treatment for cancer. She was weak, depressed and felt trapped by her situation. The first session went well – she surprised herself with what she did. She told me the next week that the morning after the previous session she woke up smiling, for the first time in months, at the memory of herself playing drums and cymbals – not the woman at all she thought herself to be!

Jung wrote 'It is not I who create myself, rather I happen to myself' (Stevens 1991). This, I think, reflects something important about the music therapy process. We do not ask a person to make consciously changes in themself. There is no analysis of problems, no interpretations of the music. Rather, through the creative musical relationship the client will often 'happen' to him or herself in a new way; will experience a different physical or emotional state along with a new quality of communication with another person.

A CREATIVE BALANCE?

Anthony Storr (1988) and Martina Thomson (1989) have both made a plea that the creative process be seen within therapy not *just* as communication: that there needs also to be a respect for the side of creating which is solitary and concerned largely with the aesthetic. The argument reflects what emphasis is placed within the different traditions of music therapy (and of arts therapies in general) on the relative importance of the intra- and inter-creative processes. In general, as would be expected, music therapists working to a psychodynamic model place greater emphasis on the client–therapist relationship whilst, at the other extreme, a therapist working to an anthroposophic model would emphasise the client's interaction with the qualities of the phenomena of the musical world.

Creative Music Therapy lies somewhere in the middle of these: acknowledging both the importance of music as communication *and* of creating music as an aesthetic experience of value for its own sake. This is perhaps nearer to how music is in our culture in general, outside of the context of the arts therapies, where there is no extra-musical agenda for the music-making (to gain access to the unconscious, to yield material for interpretation, to establish a playing relationship, etc.). The music simply works in the different ways in which music is capable: sometimes forging an intense communication between players or listeners in a relatively ephemeral improvisation; sometimes, in a more solitary process, yielding an aesthetic object which stands in its own right, and faces the creator as a whole form. That music therapy establishes a particular context for the music-making should not mean that it must narrow the richness of these different possibilities.

CHAPTER 14

Charlie

> I felt that you were with me but that you did not overcrowd my musical and therapeutic expression. The beneficial outcome for me came through a togetherness that was also intrinsically separate.

Charlie set me a challenge: musically, personally and to my ideas about music therapy. In one of our early sessions he turned round during an improvisation and told me to stop mirroring and trying to *do* something with his musical gestures:

> Surely the music isn't supposed to hold the hand of the client, it's supposed to facilitate the client maybe to do this, that, or the other. It's not necessary to save the world with your music. At this point I felt that is what you were trying to do, and it became a block for me.[1]

Charlie went on to explain that he was looking for a real musical dialogue, not just for me to be some sort of container for his musical expression. He set out other aspects of his agenda in an assessment session held at the beginning, and later in a discussion after the tenth session, when we decided whether or not to continue the work. The issues were largely concerned with the relationship between the music and the therapy. Both had been important aspects of his life until now, but had not previously come together.

---

1 Charlie's comments come (with permission from him) from those he made about the music in session 21. The reason for this is explained later.

Charlie's music therapist was Dr Colin Lee. He trained at the Nordoff-Robbins Music Therapy Centre, London in 1983. As Research Fellow in Music Therapy at City University from 1989 to 1992, he worked at London Lighthouse and was awarded his doctorate for his study of the musical significance of therapeutic improvisation. He has continued to work in palliative care.

We began working at London Lighthouse, a centre of support and services for people living with the virus HIV and AIDS which Charlie had become involved with when he was diagnosed HIV positive. He subsequently worked on the staff at Lighthouse and referred himself to music therapy. Charlie was a friendly, extrovert character who seemed well in control of himself and rarely vulnerable. Though not a trained musician he had always been involved in music, for some time in a free improvisation group. He found, however, that their rather stylised idea of improvisation did not give him the musical experience and release he felt he needed. Charlie had also tried various forms of verbal therapy and counselling, and knew how to answer a question with a question, or how to challenge me on the therapeutic aspects of the work. Most recently he had been involved in co-counselling, but found the confusion with boundaries inherent in this system could not provide him with the support he needed after he found that he had the virus.

The diagnosis had led to substantial changes in his life, though at the time we began working together he was, physically and psychologically, relatively stable. At the beginning of our work he was not afraid of telling me his needs and expectations of music therapy and that he wanted to see the sessions on four levels: (a) as music, (b) as therapy, (c) as music therapy, and (d) as words. These were, he said, separate but affiliated. The final condition was that issues of death and dying would not be discussed. I agreed to the agenda and we made an initial contract of ten sessions.

In contrast to Charlie outside music, when improvising he seemed vulnerable and chaotic, anxious, raw and at times aggressive. It was not a question of what he played, but *how*. He would push the instruments to the limit of their range – taking them apart, playing them in unconventional ways. If drums fell on the floor he would leave them there and hit them wherever they were. There was a kind of chaotic energy:

> I'm thinking here of how energy works within the whole scheme of things. That I'm putting it out, because I'm getting something out of an instrument, which has a lot of noise available in it. That sort of resonance that actually feels the way I do inside, and therefore it comes back into me. And when I hear another sound, so more comes out... The periods of wild, free playing are very important for me... I can lose control, be frenzied, and let go of all my inhibitions, be angry, violent even; it doesn't really matter what I do musically. But I don't think on the other hand that we are ever completely chaotic, I don't think we want to be. We accept the chaos in us, but we don't want to be chaotic.

The music was aleotoric in all elements: melody, harmony, rhythm and form. He resisted playing either melody or a constant pulse and had made it clear to me from the beginning that I was not to try to form this in my playing. In part his style of playing represented an anarchic intellectual and aesthetic gesture; in part it was also a way of reaching the catharsis he thought he could find in musical 'expressionism'. He spoke later that by the end of the first block of ten sessions:

> I remember feeling at this point that perhaps like the co-counselling theory – one's catharsis or discharge...if it's done through an artistic medium it can become an addiction itself. It can become patterned, and therefore it does work as a way of letting off steam, keeping us alive, but whether it shifts us in any significant direction, I wasn't sure. Maybe I was expecting too much, but if I wanted to continue with music therapy I wanted to feel assured that it was going to give me more than just an emotional discharge.

As the therapist I had also felt some sense of liberation in improvising with Charlie in a different way than is usual in music therapy sessions. And despite the sometimes self-consciously artistic intention of his improvisations Charlie would often become totally emotionally involved in his playing to the point where it *did* feel a genuine expression of his state at the time. His music gave him access to chaos in a way contrary to his everyday persona.

Charlie decided that he wanted to continue with the sessions and our evaluation of the work so far led to another agenda. The essence was that there would now be more acknowledged connection between the music and the therapy – in contrast to his earlier wish to separate out these aspects from each other. Consequently, Charlie asked that I consider the fact of his HIV status not as a separate issue but as part of the music therapy process as a whole. He seemed to want, after all, a more 'traditional' therapeutic relationship, yet one in which we were still musically equal:

> I remember thinking in retrospect how we started out. Thinking of the music and the therapy as being quite separate, and the problems that happened because of this. Then, quite unintentionally, they became joined. This is when I really began to find a personal benefit from the sessions. I felt happier about exploring areas that I would have normally held back on, due to the fact that before I felt insecure about the music therapy balance.
>
> I wanted during this period to refine our improvisations so that I could feel happy about what I could expect to happen during the session. I was beginning to feel much more exposed musically and personally,

> and so needed the safety-net of boundaries, in the sense that I was aware of a method of improvising that would encourage and not stifle what I wanted to express. I became aware that once I began to improvise, that it became a channel to let out all my own stuff, and that can be frightening. I needed to feel safe both musically and therapeutically.

There appeared to be three stages in our work. The second of these (sessions eleven to thirty) was marked by changes both in Charlie's ideas about music therapy and in the musical relationship. We found a way of playing together which suited his wish for me to have as much musical freedom as he did, but with the situation nevertheless contained within therapeutic boundaries. We became two equal but autonomous voices playing two strands of music: sometimes opposing, sometimes together. This was reflected in a broadening of the styles we played in, with a contrast between the intellectual and aleotoric idiom he started with and a style of simpler and more tonal melody which he would play on guitar, piano or tuned percussion.

There came a new level of intimacy in our musical relationship – a shared vulnerability which in turn made Charlie feel less defensive as time went on. The music, however, was not 'safe', but often had an urgent, raw quality to it. This was especially true one day when we both came into Lighthouse to find that one of the staff we both knew and liked had died, and not even from AIDS but in a senseless, accidental death. Charlie was the first client who came to me that morning, and at first we just sat, stunned. Eventually Charlie said 'I think we should just make music about this…' He happened to have his guitar with him (he brought it infrequently), and we improvised a piece for guitar and piano. His technical expertise on guitar was limited, but he made the most of a simple jazz riff and a rhythmic motif that seemed almost to cry itself. It was self-expressive but it also seemed to allow Charlie to get beyond himself in the music. The improvisation lasted about a quarter of an hour. Afterwards he left without speaking. [ʊ16]

Before we started working together Charlie had agreed to take part in the doctoral project I was then working on concerning the analysis of therapeutic improvisation. Session twenty-one was essentially the same as the others except that it was used in retrospect as part of the project. Charlie listened back to the tape of the session and selected, out of the three improvisations, the third as most clearly representing his typical musical expression at that time. This was then analysed in further depth, a process which included Charlie's verbal commentary on the musical and therapeutic aspects of the improvisation from his point of view. The details of the research are not specifically relevant here, but nevertheless both the music and Charlie's comments do very accurately represent the character of the work at this stage.

The two segments of analysis and comment represented the two characters of music we mostly played in at this time. The improvisation was on piano, four hands, with Charlie at the treble. He describes the first section:

> The music feels like I did at that time – frustrated. I didn't care, I felt hostile and angry. I wanted to express this by using the piano as a percussion instrument. I wanted to make splodges of sound, and lose any sense of trying to get things right or make good music. I remember feeling that I didn't want anything to be stable at this point, I didn't want there to be anything to hold on to. This ties in with my feelings of frustration and of feeling lost.
>
> The thing that surprises me, listening back now, is how technically good it sounds, because at the time it felt shapeless.

A musician who was another commentator on the tape described it as atonal and reminiscent of Messiaen. He heard Charlie playing clusters at the treble, whilst I anchored this with a chorale-like bass with tonal implications. A music therapist commented on the fact that 'there are aspects of individualism contained within an overall unity which is musically very beautiful'.

The second section of the improvisation (which we took as the second analysis) contrasts with the first in most respects. Again, Charlie describes:

> This section is very beautiful. I really felt as though we were sharing the most intimate feelings... A lot of this improvisation is atonal, which in a sense makes this even more tonal in feel. I'm playing a pentatonic scale and you are playing something which isn't strictly in tune with that, and yet it's in a complementary key, which when put together with my part produced breathtaking harmonies.
>
> It expressed the other side of my coin. On one hand I felt angry and annoyed. These were my first thoughts. This section made me realise that, secondary to that, but just as important, I had feelings of intimacy and pain, which we expressed through a simpler style of playing. I feel as though the rest of the improvisation was leading to this point. It works because of what had gone before.

What Charlie describes as 'atonal' was actually bitonal, with the two parts focusing on the seemingly antagonistic tonal centres of D-flat and C major. Yet the music has cohesion and invention, but within a much simpler and organised form than the musical style of the first part. This time the musician commentator said 'the two parts are so integrated with each other I can hardly believe this is an improvisation', and the other music therapist, 'the simplicity represents another side of the expression and the relationship. Both parts are separate, yet the combination of both provides a unity which is both subtle and beautiful.'

Charlie became physically quite ill at this time and emotionally seemed frightened and sometimes angry. He displayed similar reactions in the music as well – going back to his initial style of chaotic, aggressive playing. He would often, for example, spend periods of the session at the piano by himself, having wedged the sustaining pedal down with a chair, playing forceful, monolithic blocks of sound. It was quite difficult just to be beside this, and I also felt that we had lost some of the intimacy and the frequent musical contact which had become so common in the sessions before this period.

Then, quite unexpectedly, Charlie's health improved. He gained weight, began sleeping better and almost immediately the music therapy sessions changed again. This also coincided with my telling him that this would be the last six months of our work together, as I was leaving Lighthouse.

The music in this final period was more powerful than anything which had gone before, though it also went back to many of the characteristics of the point we had reached before he became ill. The musical intimacy was there again and Charlie was happy for us to play together. Something seemed to have cleared for him as a result of this period of illness. The music too had a greater clarity and intensity, though in style it was not that different from what we had played previously. There was just as much atonal and aleotoric music, but along with this was also a greater simplicity which included more sections that were sparser and tonal in design. I find it difficult to explain, but in essence it was like improvising amongst the clarity of crystal – that whilst it was never just simple, it was clear and refined, as if now we never wasted a note or phrase.

Along with this, words became less important. In essence what Charlie wanted to do was to come in, make music and go away again.

The constant questioning of the relationship between the musical content and the therapy was of central importance to Charlie – not just intellectually (as in his earlier need to set an agenda) but also in the more instinctive and creative aspects of the work. The analysis of the music we thought to be characteristic of the sessions as a whole shows above all the quality of *opposites.* This is true not just in the sense of the two opposite styles of music he played. It also comes out in the musical devices we used: bitonality, the pull of order against disorder, complex versus simple modes of expression. Also there was the sense in which Charlie found his own reconciliation of the two opposing tendencies within himself: between the expressionist giving vent to himself, and also the musician trying to get *beyond* himself and the limits of his own expression. I feel that in the last phase of the work we were able to get to this latter state together: but through a negotiation in purely musical terms which reconciled all the opposing elements, rather than from any capitulation from either of us – artistically or emotionally. The following description by Charlie of a particular moment in the music could well stand for the work as a whole:

> The power in this music lies in the fact that you did not play in the same key or mode as I did. I felt that you were with me but that you did not overcrowd my musical and therapeutic expression. The beneficial outcome for me came through a togetherness that was also intrinsically separate.

LISTENING GUIDE

[16] This longish excerpt gives the whole of the improvisation, the background to which is explained earlier in the chapter. Charlie plays guitar, the therapist piano. When listening to this it is important to remember that Charlie is untrained as a musician and self-taught as a guitarist.

CHAPTER 15

Expressing

> There exists communication between a maker and his material. We call it 'art'. There exists communication between man and man. We call it 'expression'. In this view, expression is a special case of communication and thus a possible, but not a necessary function of music. (Ernst Levy)

Notwithstanding Stravinsky's infamous remark that music is powerless to express anything at all, most people would none the less recognise an important connection between music and emotion. For centuries a philosophical and practical argument has raged over the whole issue of music and emotion: over whether music expresses, represents, arouses or contains emotion; over whether it is therefore innately therapeutic or, as Plato thought, potentially harmful.[1] A modern version of the problem has inevitably found its way into theories about, and evaluations of, the arts therapies. We often hear now that they must indeed be a good thing in that they allow people to 'express themselves'. This chapter examines some of the problems with this idea.

THE NOTION OF MUSICAL EXPRESSION

There is some confusion about the way we use the word 'expression' in everyday language. We talk of a face being expressive of anger or sadness. Yet we also 'give expression' to piano-playing, or hear expressive qualities in a performance where it is not so obviously expressive *of* anything in particular. Our common-sense recognition of expression is perhaps often

1 See 'How Music Moves' in Kivy (1990) and 'The Nature of Musical Expression' in Scruton (1983).

more apparent in its absence – whether this be in the robotic playing of a musical instrument or the dead-pan, expressionless voice of someone chronically depressed or schizophrenic.

The notion of 'expression' opens a Pandora's box which creates as many problems as it solves when trying to make sense of the arts and the arts therapies. At the same time I would emphasise that the ideas in this chapter are not an attempt to deny the role of emotion in music. On the contrary, the basic emotional involvement in music and musical communication which Creative Music Therapy gives our clients is one of its central therapeutic strengths. The problem is more a case of how the 'expressive' aspect in music and music therapy is understood.

Music therapists play regularly with people who are, as it were, on both extremes of the aesthetic argument: from people playing largely with 'feeling' but without form, whilst on the other hand those who play with form but little 'feeling'. This is an oversimplification of a complex range of musical behaviour of course, but it reflects I think a general truth. There are also theoretical positions regarding the issues of music, emotion and therapy which take a similarly polarised stance. This chapter can present just some aspects of a complex issue.

FORMS OF FEELING

In a now famous study of communication Condon and Ogston (1966) filmed conversations between mentally ill and 'normal' adults and made a microanalysis of them. One observation was of the 'flattened affect' of the ill subjects (especially those with chronic schizophrenia). They had lost in both their body and their voice what we would call the *expressive* aspects. Their bodies were semi-frozen, and failed to synchronise with the movements of the other person, and their voices had none of the *dynamic* elements which usually convey the emotional aspects of speech – the ever-varying subtleties of intensity, tone, speed, and 'melody' (also called the 'prosodic' aspects of speech). One of their conclusions was that the disturbance of self-synchrony in the ill subjects (the disynchrony in the expressive organisation of their speech and bodies) resulted in an equal failure of 'interactional synchrony', or the basic emotional rapport most healthy people experience in good communication.

Music therapist Mercedes Pavlicevic (Pavlicevic and Trevarthen 1989, Pavlicevic 1991) took the implications of this one stage further in a doctoral research project involving clinical music therapy with three contrasting groups: chronic schizophrenics, patients with unipolar depression and a group of healthy controls. Her hypothesis was influenced not just by work such as Condon and Ogston's but by the research into mother–infant interaction – so-called 'basic communication', where the aim of the interaction is primarily emotional, not one of exchanging factual information (Stern 1985). It has been observed that, in more than just a metaphorical way, the fundamental forms of emotional communication between mother and baby are *musical* ones – regardless of whether the gestures are made with the voice or the body. Mercedes Pavlicevic called these basic forms of feeling 'Dynamic Form':[2]

> The basic musical ingredients of timing, contour, dynamism, volume, timbre or texture – are a far more accurate gauge of how we are feeling than are the words that we say. When we are depressed the amount of energy in our gestures and movements decreases, and this is manifested through everything we do: gestures slow down and become sluggish, the speaking voice becomes quieter and the intonation flatter. When we are excited the converse happens: there is an increase in energy, movements are more forceful, the speaking voice is raised and its contours more animated, and we move more quickly. The dynamic features described here are musical ones, conveying to others how we are feeling. (Pavlicevic 1992)

In the same sense in which 'basic communication' is innately musical, so conversely it could be said that musical communication and interaction is innately emotional. There are indeed many similarities between mother–infant interaction and the situation of Creative Music Therapy. Both are non-verbal forms where communication, pure and simple, is the prime intention – not the transmission of new information or the creation of a self-consciously artistic piece of music. In both there is usually a 'skill-discrepancy' between the two individuals – obvious in the case of mother and baby, but also often the case in music therapy, where one player (usually the therapist) is more technically skilled in music than the client. Despite this it is nevertheless usual to succeed in establishing good interactive rapport, mostly on the basis of the shared fundamental understanding between two people of the 'Dynamic Form' of each other (the expressive gestures such as bursts of sound, halts and speed-ups, melodic swoops and rough and smooth gestures which we seem to have an innate ability to read in each other.) Pavlicevic gives the example of an infant making a floppy gesture with his

2 'Dynamic Form' is not to be confused with categorical states of emotion (e.g. anger, sadness) but with the dynamic emotional 'flow' of qualities which are perhaps the ground of the categorical states.

soft-toy which his mother models in a sound she makes with her voice. He in turn repeats his action, she repeats her sound, and with his recognition of the relationship between his action and her sound he also feels that his mother has a feeling of how he feels. So begins a mutual exploration of the relationship between feeling and form.

Similarly, Mercedes Pavlicevic describes the special form of 'clinical improvisation' used in Creative Music Therapy as 'an interface of music and "basic emotion"':

> The clinical situation of music therapy reveals the 'dynamic forms' of emotion and music at their clearest and most vivid... The 'clinical improvisation' is simply drawing out and presenting the patient's capacity for organising 'dynamic forms' in different ways, for re-creating their boundaries, for trying out new forms – within the context of a shared communicative relationship. (Pavlicevic 1992)

What happens, then, when the natural mechanisms of expressive communication and emotional rapport are disturbed by illness? The hypothesis of the experimental work in this study was that such disturbance would be highlighted in interactive musical improvisation. But also that music therapy in this approach would encourage and enhance interactive ability by working indirectly on extending and making more flexible the way a person was able to organise and share 'dynamic form' in music. These hypotheses were indeed born out by the study (Pavlicevic and Trevarthen 1989). A scale developed to rate the quality and amount of musical interaction between therapist and client showed significant differences between the three experimental groups:

> The depressed subjects conveyed coherent 'Dynamic Form'. They had not lost the capacity for some flexibility, and were able to reflect some aspects of the therapist's musical acts, despite their diminished energy and capacity to engage as fluidly and 'inter-subjectively' as the 'normal' subjects. In contrast, the schizophrenic subject's highly rigid 'Dynamic Form' prevented any meaningful interaction from taking place. (Pavlicevic 1992)

Significantly, the existence of previous musical experience of the subjects (which was accounted for in the study) did not feature as a factor in distinguishing the groups. This perhaps strengthens the argument that over and above the purely technical level of musical competence, it is rather the inherent emotional health (Winnicott's 'emotional creativity') of the person to be able to interact meaningfully which is both elicited and worked on in Creative Music Therapy. The study demonstrated statistically valid proof of improvement in these terms with the schizophrenic group in a ten-week treatment period. In short, there was an enhancement in their expressive communication as revealed in musical improvisation.

EXPRESSIONISM AND CATHARSIS

The study above demonstrates convincingly the case for the primacy of emotion in music and music therapy, and the fact that good communication (both in music and in general) can only be only be established through a flexible and reciprocal 'expressivity'. But what of the opposite scenario, when this polarity becomes an unbalanced one – where (to put it perhaps simplistically) feeling dominates form?

In a music therapy group I ran for four years (see case study in Chapter 19) I developed two simple statements which I said to the whole group every time a new member joined (these were really the only instructions I ever gave). The first was 'How you listen is more important than how you play' and the second 'You are not primarily here to express yourself!' I had, I think, positive reasons for saying the latter, but nevertheless I felt mean in the very idea of it. This was perhaps because it contradicted some people's expectations: they had come to do just this – to 'express themselves'. And this is turn is after all a perfectly reasonable expectation of an arts therapy, given how they are often presented. Since the 1960s many therapy and growth movements have championed the idea of the potential for the transformation of the self through the expression of the self. Inhibition is bad; expression of feelings healthy. As music therapy approaches also took up aspects of these ideas there came the almost unquestioned assumption that music is a straightforward expression of feelings, and therefore that one of the main functions of music therapy is to help people to express themselves through music.

A music therapist recently wrote in a professional journal, 'my training had centred on expression and catharsis' (Towse 1991). The case study presented in the article described how the client was helped to have a cathartic experience by being left alone to express herself on the instruments. ('Instruments here could be equated with a punch-bag.') There is nothing suspect in itself here – there is a now long tradition of psychotherapeutically based body-work, originating with Wilhelm Reich and others, where the intention of the therapy involves releasing blocked emotions through an expressing/purging process (whether this be hitting pillows with tennis rackets or instruments with sticks). But is there anything wrong with this?

In the music therapy group I mentioned earlier one person with the idea of 'expressing' him or herself in this particular way would often prevent the rest of the group from communicating and effectively building the music together. This was simply because someone 'expressing themself' will not, or cannot, listen to anyone else – they become trapped in a bubble of their own action and emotion. In contrast, I hope that all the case studies in this book make a strong case for the alternative view: that a vital component of improvisation and Creative Music Therapy is the quality of *listening*. This involves an inhibition of the purely self-expressive impulse in order to create a shared 'product' together. All this can sound perilously like a prescriptive form of denial. Yet I believe it is actually a help within the music therapy situation. It is not denying the basic emotional content of music and music therapy, but countering the theoretical *idea* that cathartic expression of feeling is all there is to it.

The last point is a vital one. The above is not to invalidate the evidence of the first section which emphasises the basic, necessary expressive component of music in communication. What I am questioning, on the contrary, is rather a concept of expression – a culturally formed notion called 'expressionism' which has become an everyday notion in our times, whether in art or personal conduct. The 'expressionist' believes in the need not just for emotional immediacy but that this needs to be consciously 'expressed' (the origin of the word coming from the Latin, meaning 'to force out'). He also believes that any outer form (be this our bodies or our art) is a direct expression of an 'inner content'. In short that what we do, what we make, is how we are.

SELF-EXPRESSION AND ARTISTIC FORM

At one level, of course, all this is true. Expressing your pain, joy or sadness is part of a basic human instinct of immediate and spontaneous emotional reaction. It involves a simple correlation between the internal state and the external form of the expression. If I stub my toe I usually scream: the intensity of the pain equates directly with the scream. The problem comes when this everyday experience becomes converted into a theory of what 'should' happen in art or therapy, and in turn into a prescriptive doctrine. For both art and the art therapies are more than simply 'expressing yourself'. As the philosopher Suzanne Langer wrote: 'Sheer self-expression requires no artistic form... Music is not self-expression, but formulation and representation of emotions, moods, mental tensions and resolutions – a "logical picture" of sentient, responsive life, a source of insight not a plea for sympathy' (Langer 1960). A client came to me for individual music therapy and told me that this was how she needed to express herself. The first session she assaulted the percussion instruments with vigour and commitment for half an hour. Throughout this time I was attempting to play with her on the piano, using every trick in my book to give her the hint that we were playing *together*. When I later listened to the tape of the sessions I could hardly hear the piano, so loud and insistent was the percussion. She remained for this session and most of the next firmly in the cocoon of her self-expression (though admittedly reporting that she felt better afterwards). Gradually, however, the fury abated and we started to find a musical dialogue between us: to listen and respond to each other. Her music did not lose its fire, but what became important in the therapy for her was not her initial idea of expressing herself but of being responded to in the music. She called it 'having a resonance'. Feeling was still first, but it was her *ideas* about feeling and music, and what the music therapy process should be, that got in the way at first.

Another example comes from the comment I have quoted before from a client of a colleague: 'It's fascinating. When I think about expressing myself I hear only my inner gesture coming out. When I listen to the music it's terrifying, because I hear the two of us meeting.'

We all start from the point of expressing ourselves: presenting ourselves the only way we can, trapped more or less in our own bubble. But what most of us try to do, and what it is the therapist's job to help people with, is to get beyond this bubble of self: to create something new in ourselves through a dialogue with someone or something beyond ourselves. As Karl Popper writes:

> The expressionist believes that all he can do is to let his talent, his gifts, express themselves in his work. The result is good or bad according to the mental or physiological state of the worker. As against this I suggest that everything depends upon the give-and-take between ourselves and our work; upon the *product* which we contribute. (Popper 1976)

EXPRESSION OR EXPLORATION

In the epigraph to this chapter, Ernst Levy (Levarie and Levy 1983) made the distinction between 'art' as 'the communication between a maker and his material', and 'expression' as 'communication between man and man'. Most people would agree with the observation that art-works are not *necessarily* self-expressive in any direct way. It is also true, however, that the improvised dialogue which is the basis of Creative Music Therapy is not the same as a crafted composition. The improvisation is more immediate, unpredictable and bodily. Nevertheless I would still argue that an improvisation in music therapy is closer in spirit to the composer's imaginative and creative process than it is to the cathartic 'musical scream' of a person instinctively expressing their anger on a drum.

In Creative Music Therapy there is, even at the simplest level, this give-and-take both between the client and the music, and between the client and therapist through the music. The dialogue we have with the material or other people in making something new in the world is an exploration of our thought and feeling, not just a simple expression. We make something out of experience and feeling, using our in built capacity to give experience form through symbol and metaphor.

Improvised musical dialogue has its life *between* the personal worlds of two or more people: as a totally authentic creation of both of us, whilst being a purely personal 'self-expression' of neither of us. I used to tell the music therapy group mentioned earlier to imagine that the music they were improvising came from the middle of the ceiling – that while everyone in the room was indispensable to what happened, no single person was responsible for it – that in a way it was playing them. By actively working on listening, responding and creating within the music, instead of expressing ourselves something else happened: the process of 'meeting', creating and communicating in the music.

One of the strengths and delights of musical improvisation is its mercurial flow of emotional resonance, the range of its 'musical territory'. Even a relatively short stretch of music can contain a gamut of musical idioms, tempos, textures, 'feelings'. On the contrary, having *ideas* about how music relates to emotions tends in fact to limit what it can do. A person who has decided to play 'sad' music artificially forces this idea on the playing and limits it to just that. The issue becomes even more wrong-headed when certain categorical 'musical moods' are 'prescribed' to create a certain effect in a person. As Peter Kivy (1990) points out, 'sad' music no more makes us genuinely sad than watching *Hamlet* makes us suicidal! On the contrary, as Suzanne Langer has written:

> Music can present emotions and moods we have *not* felt, passions we did *not* know before. It's subject matter is the same as that of 'self-expression', and its symbols may be borrowed, on occasion, from the realms of expressive symptoms; yet the borrowed elements are *formalised*, and the subject matter 'distanced' in an artistic perspective. (Langer 1960)

Many of our clients in music therapy are stuck in habitual physical and psychological states. One of the gifts of active music-making as a dialogue is that they often find themselves experiencing different and unpredicted new feelings, thoughts and experiences: not ones that have been pre-planned or 'prescribed' to lead to catharsis, or indeed any specific effect.

A client of mine came into her session recently in a mood of self-dramatic hopelessness, determined not to care what she played or how she played it. She began to play a drum with a careless, brushing movement. I improvised music to match at first, but gradually and inevitably the music changed into something quite different – a graceful waltz. The conflict was visible and audible, between the *idea* of the mood she wanted to hold on to, and the actual feeling in the music and her changing style of playing which, because of her musicality, she could not help living. I am glad to say the music won!

CONCLUSION

Perhaps Levy's attempt to tease out 'art' and 'expression' will not do in the end. Music is neither pure feeling nor pure form, and this is also true in the music therapy situation. One of the lessons music therapy has to offer the more refined worlds of musicology and aesthetics is just how rooted music is in the body. The 'expressive' elements of music are fundamentally related to the communicative grammars of our bodies, a fact that can be seen when these are interfered with by illness. It is because of this dynamic relationship between music, communication and expression that music therapy can work so powerfully.

Creative Music Therapy is able to meet the client on the level of both form and feeling. The therapist may indeed start by matching the expressive gestures of the client. But when the musical relationship progresses the dialogue leads both to the point where they can also let the music 'feel for itself', where the purely musical world frees us from our purely personal world.

If we keep in mind that the essential process of therapy is a journey rather than a statement, then it becomes important how music can act to allow people to discover themselves creatively, as both form *and* feeling. The 'musical product' which is between people making music together works like a magic mirror – it reflects back to the players physical and emotional vistas they have not felt before.

CHAPTER 16

Jack

> If they are to have what 'he' has just done then I should think they would be very happy.

One Tuesday afternoon Jack came for the first time to the music therapy unit. His appointment followed that of Dominic, a seven-year-old autistic boy who held my hand as I took him back to his mother in the waiting room. Jack had come with his wife, and said politely, 'Pleased to meet you' when she introduced us. Then, just like Dominic, Jack took my hand and let me lead him into the therapy room. There continued to be strange parallels between Jack and Dominic throughout this time: one a child yet to find a self, the other a man of sixty-five whose self threatened to disintegrate, and whose behaviour had become child-like.

His wife told me that Jack had begun to show signs of Alzheimer's disease as long as ten years ago, but that he had deteriorated rapidly in the last year and now needed constant care. He had a puzzling pattern of both damage and ability: often confused over the simplest things yet sometimes making apposite jokes and enjoying listening to the radio and watching *Mastermind* on television.

Jack was an immediately likeable man, gentle and dignified despite the indignities his illness inflicted on him. He had been a respected teacher and was an educated and cultured man. His passions were music and cricket (the latter turning out to be more significant in his music therapy than might be expected).

Jack seemed lost and anxious when he got into the music therapy room, so I asked him to sit beside me at the piano. The piano had been recently polished and Jack happened to be sitting at a level where he could see his reflection in the piano lid (though I did not realise this at the time).

> 'How often do you let them out?' asked Jack.

> 'Sorry, Jack?'
>
> 'How often do you let them out – the people in the piano?', he repeated.

'Oh, at least twice a day', I said, thinking quickly, not wanting to cut across his world so soon – then seeing why he had made such a bizarre comment. Jack was quite happy with my answer. In the early sessions he would talk quite a lot, perhaps out of anxiety, and it often seemed a jumble of surreal connections. But I learned to listen more carefully as we went on, for under the seeming nonsense he was frequently saying something relevant and significant, though often in a euphemistic and poetic way.

I gave Jack a side drum and a cymbal with one beater, but he had no idea what to do with them. I showed him and encouraged him to play:

> 'Go on Jack...have a go!'
>
> 'I'm not sure...put it on, then, and we'll see how it goes [looking at his drumstick] you know, I think I need a curved one of these!'

On the piano I played simple music with a clear beat, but Jack was wary of playing. He appeared, though, to be listening to the music, and began to tap his other hand with the drumstick.

> 'Try on the drum now Jack...'

He began to play the drum in a regular, careful beat, but around the rim, not on the skin. He then found the centre and the proper sound of the drum and, looking pleased with himself, commented in one of his characteristic cricketing metaphors:

> 'I bowled that one straight down the line.'

There was seldom any continuity in Jack's playing and my job was to somehow get him inside the music so that *it* could involve and stabilise him. [ʊ17]

Though getting Jack to play was often a problem he invariably seemed to listen carefully, and often complemented me on what I played: 'You've got a quick hand there' he'd say. When we did manage to play together there was a definite contact between us in the music, if only sporadically. If, however, I made the music too complex or changed it too quickly I lost him.

Instead of changing the style of music too much I tried changing the instrument and gave Jack a xylophone with just the black notes, giving a simple pentatonic mode I thought would not be too complicated for him.

> 'I'm quite excited by this!' said Jack.
>
> 'Good. Have a play!'

But again he had no idea how to use the instrument, and my idea of the simplified pentatonic arrangement back-fired. He managed (quite skilfully) to play not the notes, but the cracks between the notes, making a nasty wooden sound. As usual he had a strangely apposite comment:

> 'That one went off again!'

Sitting with me at the piano and playing the black notes at the top Jack managed a more shaped melody, but this was hampered by his appealing for inspiration to an imaginary person behind us. I thought it was probably time to stop. Given his condition Jack had both concentrated and persevered for a surprisingly long time.

> 'I'll come back again. I'll be back up here again', he said as we (confusingly) walked *up* the stairs from the crypt.

Jack was more relaxed when he came the next time, and there were longer stretches of consistent playing, partly because I was finding the kind of music he needed; simple melody and phrasing, clear harmony, 'quickening' rhythm and repetitive structures. Waltzes, hornpipes and simple classical styles seemed to engage him. His playing (on drums, cymbal and tambourine) became more extended and he began sometimes to initiate the music. In these times Jack was involved and animated and, as he concentrated on the music, there were fewer verbal interruptions. That is, until he suddenly said:

> 'It's not as good as it should be...but what can I do to alter this?'

In his life Jack had been something of a perfectionist, and it seemed a cruel twist of fate that now, in his disability, he was still aware of the gap between what he thought he should do and what he could do. His wife had talked of his frustration, and it seemed that this was now entering into our music therapy sessions. Jack was still setting himself standards of achievement. He continued:

> 'I feel as if I can really get going if I can come back to you...I'll be back as quick as I can...I'm very pleased in some places, but absolutely appalled in others. I've really enjoyed it so far.'

His last statement was encouraging. At least there was enjoyment, not just the feeling of yet another task which he could do less well than he wanted.

In the next few sessions there was certainly more awareness and involvement from Jack. He still needed encouragement to start anything, but the playing that followed had more coherence. His playing on the black notes of the piano flowered unexpectedly into melody. He liked the gently syncopated music I improvised to his playing of the bongos, which started tentatively but, as usual with Jack, suddenly 'found' an involvement and coherence.

> 'Getting more confident' he assured me, but then: 'Do you think I'll get anywhere?'

I knew by now that this was a hint that frustration was setting in, and that it would be wise to go on to another activity. But he preempted me by asking:

> 'What would you do if you met a girl?'

Even for Jack, this was an unusual connection, and I replied in keeping:

> 'Oh, I'd sing to her...'

I improvised a song, hoping that it might encourage Jack to sing himself, something he had never done with me before. He was amused by my singing but did not join in. Would a song he recognised be better, I wondered, and tried 'Ye banks and ye braes'. But it seemed even less effective – the inflexibility of a song in comparison to improvisation failed to catch his attention.

Jack's wife watched the next session. In one sense it cannot have been much comfort for her to see the man she once knew as dignified and cultured now playing a drum with childish glee. But in another sense she said it was very moving. In the last two years he had progressively lost his ability to concentrate or get involved in any activity and to communicate effectively with another person. And, along with the loss of these, he had also lost any sense of enjoyment and achievement. 'The quality of his life is so low usually' she said. What she saw in the music therapy session was the restoration of some quality in Jack's life: his sustained attention and positive engagement in his playing, his ability to share an activity with another person, and a decrease of the frustration, confusion and delusions that dogged his everyday life. But it was also true that many of these qualities were only evident while the music lasted, though she reported (as have other therapists) that the increased sense of integration lasted for several hours after the end of the session. What moved his wife was simply how happy he looked in the best moments of the music-making.

This was nicely illustrated the day Jack found a horn on top of the piano. I had been using a shiny silver one-note horn with Dominic in the session before – the ideal thing to catch a child's attention. It also caught Jack's eye, and when I gave it to him he blew it loudly (in contrast to the soft, tentative way he approached any other instrument).

> 'We'll wake everything up!' said Jack.

I found a second horn, tuned to another note to play myself, and we began a playful dialogue on the two horns, experimenting with long and short notes, and horn-like rhythmic motifs. Almost unlike any other music we had played together this had such musical meaning, and such human meaning between us. But most of all we were having such fun. Jack laughed and said 'That was good!' [☊18] As we were leaving the room at the end of the session he said:

> 'You know, this is the best thing of this kind that I do!'

Alzheimer's disease is remorseless in its progression and it became obvious that music therapy too had its limits. We managed about twenty sessions together, but it became increasingly stressful both for Jack and the people who cared for him to get him to the unit. The problems eventually outweighed the benefits and we reluctantly agreed to stop.

What remains with me, however, is a comment that Jack made at the end of his penultimate session. We had walked back to meet his wife in the waiting room where there were on that day a large number of people waiting to see the doctor. Jack often referred to himself in the third person and, looking at all the people, he turned to me and said:

> 'If they are to have what "he" has just done then I think they would be very happy.'

LISTENING GUIDE

[☊17] The therapist plays a simple eight-bar melody whilst Jack looks somewhat lost sitting in front of a side-drum by the side of the piano, the beater resting on the drum. 'Here's your stick' the therapist says, giving it to Jack. 'I won't be able to pick up that' he replies (meaning the music, I think, not the stick), but in fact does this straight away – first playing a simple pulse to the music, then some of the melodic rhythm of the tune. At the end of the second repetition he loses either his concentration or his confidence and his beat falters. 'I missed that one!' he says.

[☊18] In this excerpt we use two 'reed horns', specially designed to produce with relative ease just one tone. Jack plays the higher of the two (E), the therapist a horn tuned a fifth lower (A). At first he is confused about how to play and the therapist demonstrates, at the beginning of this excerpt, with a long 'A' (also playing the piano with just the left hand) and encourages Jack to play. He tentatively begins on the higher tone, then becomes more confident, playing both long tones and short rhythmic motifs. This soon leads into an energetic dialogue between the two horns.

CHAPTER 17

Recalling

> It happened that Lucy, who found daily life rather chaotic, entered a more solid world when she opened the piano. (E.M. Forster, *A Room With a View*)

Music has often been characterised as a wordless call – the Orpheus legends and the Siren's song being archetypal images of music's power. Music therapy also makes use of this capacity of music to reach down into a person's consciousness when words and other means of contact have failed.

Related to the idea of music as call is that of 'recall'; of how the order of music can recall a sense of order when the self is threatened by the chaos of the external world or from the disordering effects of illness or handicap. As it did for Lucy, the character in E.M. Forster's novel, music can often provide a more solid world than does everyday reality.

Disintegration, disorder, disconnection – these have always been descriptive of illness, whilst their opposites – integration, order and connection – are, as Oliver Sacks has remarked, the necessary qualities of any therapy, 'One way of "centring", of recalling a self, the active powers of a self, from the abyss of pathology, can be given by music, by art of all kinds' (Sacks 1991).

This chapter considers music acting to call and to 'recall' within the music therapy situation, and how these functions may be connected to an essential characteristic of music in general.

BELOW CONSCIOUSNESS – MUSIC THERAPY WITH COMA PATIENTS

Dagmar Gustorff's work in Germany with people in coma is perhaps the most dramatic use of music as call.[1] Many of the clients we see in music therapy are in some way isolated physically or emotionally, but none so critically as the person in coma. These people experience profound psycho–physical disorientation in space and time, their 'centre' of consciousness lost. The situation is sometimes compounded, as was shown in the case of Herr G., by the confusing noise of an intensive care unit and the attempts of staff and relatives to communicate by shouting instructions to the patient.

In contrast to this was the quiet singing of the music therapist, who sang not just *to* the patient, but attempted to relate the music to how he was at that time – taking, at minimum, his breathing rhythm and heartbeat 'into' the music. The exact procedure was described earlier in Herr G.'s case, and rather than repeat this I want to look at some of its implications.

Dagmar Gustorff's work with coma patients came about as an unexpected development from working with a man with a neurological condition. When he was too ill to come to music therapy sessions he asked if she would still work with him, and this continued until he went into coma. The therapist, not wanting to desert him at this point, then found that even though he was unconscious she could still be with him musically by singing to him in the particular way she developed. Herr G.'s own report confirms that there was a qualitative difference between how he experienced the music in comparison to the other more desperate attempts to communicate with him in words. The music gave him both a sense of human contact and an orientation in his disconnected and at times hallucinatory world:

> The point it all changed was when I first heard the music...the music was exquisite! The first time I didn't recognise it as a voice, but as some kind of mediaeval wind instrument. But the second time I knew it was a voice, that there was a person there, there was someone who didn't want to kill me. I remember thinking 'there *is* life, there is something else but this, there is someone who wants me to survive...and not only wants me, but is helping me to connect to life again'. The music I felt was *my* music. I decided to live when I first heard the music.

Dramatic though the circumstances of this case were, the music therapy work was not fundamentally different in principle from the other case studies in this book – where aspects of the musical experience allow a contact to be made between people when often other mediums have failed. It is also clear from Herr G.'s case that music is not just being made *for* him but that, as in a more conventional music therapy relationship, he also has a way of

---

1 See the case history, Herr G. in Chapter 7. Music therapists in England also work with clients in coma or persistent vegetative states (see Bunt 1994).

responding musically – if only in 'phrased breathing'. The scheme I proposed earlier in this book for describing musical relationship (see Chapter 8) holds good, I think, for this work with an unconscious client. Both a therapist improvising with a client playing a drum and one singing to the breathing of a comatose patient are doing much the same thing, and giving much the same experience to the client – that he is being met in the music and accompanied in his isolation.

During the short music therapy sessions the reactions of the comatose patients ranged from a change in breathing (becoming slower and deeper) to fine motor movements of the head and hands, to in some cases them opening their eyes and regaining consciousness. At the beginning of the singing the heart rate slowed down, then rose rapidly, sustaining this elevated level for the duration of the session. EEG measurements of brain activity show a desynchronisation from theta rhythm to alpha or beta in former synchronised areas. In a paper looking at the implications of this work, David Aldridge (1991) interprets these physiological data as indicating 'arousal and perceptual activity...and an attempt at orientation and cognitive processing within the communicational context':

> We can speculate that the various body rhythms have become disassociated in comatose states and following major surgery. The question remains of how these behaviours can be integrated and where the seat of such integration is. It is quite clear that integration is an organisational property of the whole organism in relationship with the environment and not located in any one organ. The environment of the patient includes the vital component of human contact, and there is reason to believe that the essential ground of this contact too is rhythmical. (Aldridge 1991)

RECALLING A SELF

Music can therefore function both as call and 're-call', where it acts to help re-integrate a person's perceptions and overall consciousness. For most of us our identity and feeling of security in the world comes from the reliability and continuity of those perceptions of space and time which underpin both our physiological and psychological life. But this very security can be radically undermined by illness – coma being the most extreme, but by no means the only example. In order to understand people in this situation and to be able to develop appropriate help we need, as Oliver Sacks has written, an 'existential neurology...a neurology of the self, in dissolution and creation' (Sacks 1990, 1991). From both his personal and professional experience Sacks recommends music and art as means to orientate and integrate the self. In *Music and the Mind* Anthony Storr suggests how this might be possible in the case of music:

> Music can order our muscular system. I believe that it is also able to order our mental contents. A perceptual system originally designed to inform us of spatial relationships by means of imposing symmetry can be incorporated and transformed into a means of structuring our inner world. (Storr 1992)

In previous case studies we have seen how the music worked to lend its energy, movement or 'feeling' to the client. How, then, does music manage to give this sense of order and integration to people like Jack? Is there a specific ordering property of music? On the contrary, it would seem as if this time we are dealing not with a separate element of music but a characteristic of it as a whole – how it orders itself within its own parameters of space and time. And though perhaps this aspect of music is needed most by those whose integration is threatened, most people none the less find the sense of order and the intimations of wholeness in music a major factor in their need for it, either as players or listeners.

THE TIME AND SPACE OF MUSIC

St. Augustine remarked that he knew what time was until he tried to explain it. Similarly, philosophers and psychologists of music have focused in on this aspect, characterising music as 'the art of time' or its effect as a 'shaping of time'.[2] Zuckerkandl (1973) remarked that music is not just in time, but that it does something *with* time. Stravinsky followed his famous sentence about music being powerless to express anything with a second clause (usually omitted in quotation), that 'the phenomenon of music is given to us with the sole purpose of establishing an order in things, particularly the coordination between Man and Time' (Stravinsky 1947).

Most people experience music as having somehow its own time and space – where these are qualitatively different from the time of the clock and the space of the map. It is commonplace that people often talk of being 'lost' during the time of music. But there is also another important quality of 'musical time': that a piece often feels both complete as a form whilst at the same time it continues unfolding something more and something new in the time you are listening (or playing). Moreover, when the music is improvised

---

2 See 'Toward the Phenomenology of Music' in Dahlhaus (1982).

rather than being a pre-planned and notated composition this effect is even more striking. The music takes form and weaves together the time of its performance even though it is being created on the point of that present. This 'organic unity' of music gives it a quality different from the other arts, and therefore a potentially unique quality for music therapy.

A television documentary was shown a few years ago called *Prisoner of Consciousness* about the professional choral conductor Clive Wearing who fell victim to a devastating neurological condition which resulted in him being stranded in the present. His recent past became obliterated every couple of minutes, though he retained a tragic awareness of his problem since he continually 'woke up'. 'It's like being dead all the time' he said as he paced anxiously around the room in the psychiatric unit he then had to stay in. Though he retained some basic facts about his life (that he was married and had children), he seemed to have little personal connection to this information – it no longer gave him a sense of identity.

Three scenes in the film showed one of the few things which could recall him into wholeness, dignity and integration – his participation in music. In the first of these Clive Wearing was taken back to the chapel of his old Cambridge college and, seated at the organ, said 'I'm so rusty, it's the first time I've seen this' (it was not, of course), 'What am I supposed to do?' He then proceeded to play fluently and well, though soon afterwards had already forgotten about it. In another scene he went back to the choir he had conducted professionally only a few years previously. Again, after initial confusion, the music seemed to recall his powers of concentration, involvement and professionalism. He then asked where he was and who all the people were. The third excerpt showed him in a more comfortable situation, without perhaps the unnecessarily dramatic set-ups. This time he was at home in his room playing Bach on the harpsichord for himself. He played by memory and, significantly, the length of the piece was considerably longer than the extant length of his memory span. His wife reflected that the two things which recalled him to wholeness were music and love.

In one sense these musical situations were recalling Clive Wearing back to his sense of identity and ability as a musician and giving him a rare window into his past. But this is not quite everything – these performances were not just the comfort of memory. His *living* involvement with the music, playing Bach or conducting a motet, were fully of the present. Whilst his illness involved the *dis*-continuity of time, music gave him the opposite experience – an integration and inter-penetration of time moments. The same phenomenon was apparent in my work with Jack and has been reported by other music therapists working with people with neurological conditions – particularly Alzheimer's Disease (Aldridge and Aldridge 1992).

THE FLOW OF MUSIC

The physicist David Bohm used the phenomenology of music to illustrate the elusive processes of quantum mechanics:

> Consider, for example, how music is comprehended. At any given moment, a particular note may be sounding in awareness, but at the same time, a kind of 'reverberation' of a number of earlier notes can also be sensed. Such reverberation is not the same as recollection or memory. Rather it is more like part of an unbroken enfoldment and unfoldment of the notes concerned into even subtler forms, including emotions and impulses to physical movement, as well as a kind of ethereal echo of the original notes within the mind. Indeed if successive notes are played several seconds apart, they no longer combine together in such a way as to convey the dynamic sense of unbroken flow. This suggests that, at any given moment, a number of notes are present in awareness in various degrees of enfoldment. The simultaneous awareness of these is what constitutes the sense of unbroken flow. (Bohm and Peat 1989)

It is unlikely, however, that any of this could be reduced to a purely physical explanation. Whilst there can be a physics of sound perception, hearing music is to hear musical *meaning*, where the parts are connected to an ongoing whole by the intentional activity of the mind. And this involves not just a way of hearing but real and active properties of the music itself. For example, a melody is a structure which connects together in a subtle hierarchy – according to acoustic, musical and cultural conventions. Each tone is not separate but contains a 'force' (both melodic and harmonic) which gives it direction towards and connection to the next tone. Groups of tones then organise themselves into motifs and phrases, which are themselves 'nested' within larger phrases and periods. A similar hierarchy of organisation could be traced for each of the components of music.

Zuckerkandl (1973) suggests that the logic of music is really not adequately described by the past–present–future delineation everyday logic gives us. Rather, musical logic starts in the middle, as it were, giving the experience of a present unfolding both backwards and forwards, rather like Figure 17.1.

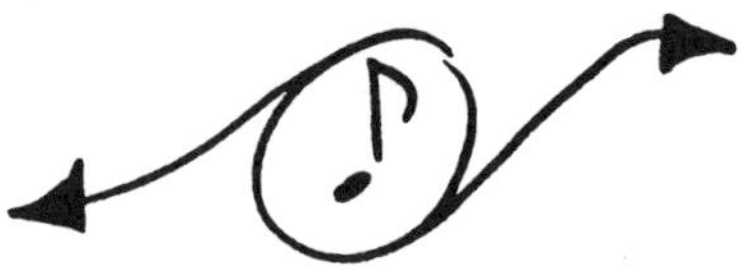

Figure 17.1

Zuckerkandl explains:

> Those who, by means of the grammatical tenses, divide time into different kinds of time put themselves outside of time, let time flow by. But to hear music is to be flowing with time, is to know the past and the future only as characteristics of the flowing present, as its two directions, away from and toward. (Zuckerkandl 1973)

Perhaps it is this integrated *flow* of music that best describes not only the subject of this chapter but also other phenomena of the music therapy experience: the physical flow and motivation I have called 'quickening'; the flow of creativity; the flow of 'feeling'. In each case the flow and integration of music is a compensation for the scattered, the incoherent and the discontinuous.[3]

The man who, in Oliver Sacks' famous case, 'mistook his wife for a hat' would continually sing songs in order to retain the connection between his actions and the objects which were continually losing their meaning and function for him. Without his eating, dressing and bathing songs he would simply lose the thread of things and come to a stop. Sacks comments, 'I think that music, for him, had taken the place of image. He had no body-image, he had body-music: that is why he could move and act as fluently as he did, but came to a confused stop if the "inner music" stopped' (Sacks 1985).

THE MUSIC OF MEMORY

This is not to forget the more everyday connection between music and memory, which ranges from pleasant nostalgia to powerful 'Proustian' recollections spurred by music. Musical memory establishes connections and resonances both within an ongoing piece and associatively within our long-term memory. In his account of his depressive illness, *Darkness Visible*, the American novelist William Styron (1992) cites the turning point for him as a chance hearing of a fragment of Brahms' *Alto Rhapsody* on the soundtrack

3 See also Czikszentmihalyi's (1988, 1992) characterisation of 'flow' as 'optimal experience'.

of a video. This reminded him of his mother singing this same piece and set in train a series of thoughts and feelings which averted him from acting on his wish to take his life. The connections which the music made broke thought the closed circle of his psychological state.

For clients in Creative Music Therapy aspects of musical memory are equally important. In her work with Herr G. Dagmar Gustorff used just a single melodic phrase, repeated both within and between the sessions. Herr G. later remarked that he recognised this phrase when he was in coma, and it must have been one of the few impressions he was able to hold on to in that state – and one of the few things which made any connection in his disorientation. In my work with Emanuella it was the resonances of the musical style which gave some depth to her musical experience, linking it to earlier family and cultural memories. With Tom also, the songs which were the 'leitmotivs' in his music therapy connected him to his family and a time when he had a sense of identity in the family skiffle band.

For the music therapist the challenge is to ensure that this musical memory works to add something to the present situation, not to trap people in the past. It is all too easy for nostalgia to become empty repetition, or that a person shuts themself away in their self-contained and safe musical time-capsule, avoiding a creative musical relationship in the present. Improvisation is a great help here. It can side-step the dangers of inflexible repetition and can take the familiar (a melody or idiom) as a starting-point and then develop into the less familiar. This keeps the music and the musical relationship living whilst still resonating with the positive qualities of musical memory.

CHAPTER 18

Tom

> Music is a memory bank for finding one's way about the world. (Bruce Chatwin)

The 'songlines' which Bruce Chatwin describes in his book are both a form of map and an ancestral memory-bank which the Aborigines use to orientate themselves in their sacred territory. Tom also used songs to orientate himself, but for him this was more of a question of time – where the songs helped him retrieve the security of the past when present anxiety threatened him.

Tom came to music therapy already with his own seemingly complete musical world. I found out that he had played percussion for the family skiffle band for much of his life, and consequently had a repertoire of songs and a strong idea of just how the music should go. Unlike most clients in their first session, Tom was quite at home with the situation, arranged the percussion instruments, selected the right sticks and was away!

Playing in the skiffle band represented the secure part of Tom's life, where he had been looked after by his family. After the death of his mother, however, he had moved into a community for adults with learning difficulties. The other fascination in his life apart from music was trains, and perhaps the caricature image of the train-spotter is the best simple description of him. He was fifty-one when I first met him: a large man with a mass of neat greying curly hair. He seemed easy-going and amiable, with a friendly earnestness. His speech was hard to understand both because of a stammer and a strange abbreviated syntax he used, where selected key-words served as whole sentences.

Cheow Godfrey worked with Tom at the Marylebone Music Therapy Unit in London. She is currently developing a music therapy project with adults with special needs in London.

Verbal communication was one of Tom's frustrations, but there were obviously others. His keyworker, who had searched out music therapy as a possible help for Tom, explained that over the last few years the frustration and bottled-up emotions seemed to be getting worse, with Tom being uncharacteristically difficult at home. One of the stranger signs of his distress was when he would blacken his face with earth. Evidently this referred back to his childhood when his family lived beside a coal-mine. Tom seemed to associate both his distress and his 'bad' behaviour with the blackened face of the miners.

Tom had firm ideas about what music we should be playing in the sessions, and what my role would be in this. For the first six months or so Tom played 'his' music – complex flurries of drum and cymbal which, though creative in the actual use of the instruments, was both unvarying in style and pace and, more importantly, largely uncommunicative musically. I had the impression at this stage that Tom's music was less an event in the present than an accompaniment to something in the past going on in his head – perhaps a re-run of playing in the family skiffle-band. He seemed largely unaware of what was actually happening in the present; either what I played on the piano along with his drumming, or even I suspect what he himself was doing. It was not really very creative, more like playing a recording to himself.

Tom's music also included his repertoire of songs, of which there were three favourites: the *6–5 Special*, the *Hallelujah Song* and the *Come Along Song*. These seemed to represent either important times or the important subjects of his life: some his childhood and the skiffle-band, whilst the *6–5 Special* came from a television programme about trains. In one sense I felt these were like totems of security to him, and this was apparent in how Tom used them within the music therapy sessions at moments of insecurity or disorientation. But he also, I suspect, played the songs simply because he liked them and because this was the only time in the week where somebody was there to listen and play them with him. At the beginning I had few illusions as to what Tom expected of me – I was there to help him play the songs!

This situation led, however, to two rather opposing intentions about what should be happening in the sessions. Tom, for his part, was happy and determined to continue in his style, with its jazz-style drumming, taking refuge in one of his beloved songs at any opportunity. On the other hand, my attempts to encourage Tom to play different music in other ways simply became a resistance to what he wanted to do. It was an impasse, and I felt frustrated after six months or so of this – it seemed we played only our own music, rather than any music we shared between us. The further what I played was away from Tom's preferred style, the quicker he took refuge in the songs. I even tried deviously avoiding them altogether for a time, which led to the predictable result – the more I avoided them, the more they became part of the session, but in a negative way.

At this stage I thought again about the whole situation and decided to try the opposite approach regarding the songs – going along with them, but with the intention of developing them between us, rather than just reproducing them as frozen forms. This was largely successful – sometimes we would play the songs simply and intact (still of course the way he liked them best), but gradually I introduced other ways of playing the songs. I would, for example, sometimes play only an accompanying bass-line, so that Tom had to sing the tune himself. Other times I would slow the songs down, speed them up, change them into the relative major or minor key and so on, each time using these variations as a spring-board for free improvisation.

This approach was at first, as you can imagine, far from popular with Tom. But he gradually came round to both accepting it and enjoying it. As he learned to trust me more he also allowed me to take these liberties with his precious songs. But equally, through my acceptance of his songs he came to accept me and what I had to offer musically. Through this symbolic tolerance of each other we also arrived at a new level of playing, where there was far more of a mutual give and take in the music. Tom always retained much of his preferred style of playing, but there was also an important difference in the situation – his playing was not always within the closed bubble of himself (and possibly also the past). We were now mostly playing *together* in a real sense, influencing each other in the here and now of the music. With this I felt I was meeting Tom at a much deeper level in the music.

There had been times when Tom would start talking in the session seemingly to avoid playing in a different style, or when I gave him an instrument that was not his favoured drum and cymbal combination. The talking stopped, however, except for occasional comments about what we were doing, especially if he liked it. But one puzzling aspect of the work was the way in which Tom seemed to find little enjoyment in any improvisation with a melodic element which did not involve the songs. I would offer Tom the xylophone to play, but I often felt that he played it as a favour to me rather than because he found any satisfaction in it. He tended to play melodic instruments in a rhythmic rather than a melodic way, with little attention to phrasing or melodic expression. This seemed paradoxical in relation to the almost talismanic power the melodic identity of the songs held for him. It was almost as if melody was 'outside' of him, not something which he produced as an expression of himself. I had the strange hunch that if Tom could really play a melody he would somehow be whole: that melody represented the other side to the frenetic drumming and his frustration and isolation. The work with the songs was perhaps the beginning of this transition, but it was slow and ongoing work.

Of the anger and outbursts, which had been one of the reasons for referring Tom to music therapy in the first place, I have seen no sign and suspect I never will. The context we work in is very different from the situation where Tom became upset and angry. The music therapy sessions were an island in his world where he felt fulfilled and accepted. After working together for two years the home where Tom lived reported that the worst of the problem seemed to have passed.

Previously Tom used either the positive symbols of his songs or the negative ones of his face-blackening gesture to shore up his sense of self. But both of these referred back, were somehow stuck outside his present reality. In contrast, I think that Tom's sense of himself changed through his work in music therapy and that he retained this feeling to an extent outside the session. Tom was still different 'inside' and 'outside' music, but there was more movement between these extremes, in the same way as in our improvisations there was a progression from the habitual and repetitive to something creative and living. Music was a very physical thing to Tom – it gave him a real sense of being; it was when he took on his most vivid look. Tom 'outside' of music is Tom somehow displaced – he doesn't seem to fit in. But when Tom is 'inside' music, everything fits together.

CHAPTER 19

The Wednesday Group

> Composed music says 'I'; improvised music says 'We'. The improviser listens primarily to the people improvising with him. The improviser is part of a community. (Joachim-Ernst Berendt)

'Music is a social fact' concluded the ethnomusicologist John Blacking after having experienced and studied many musical cultures. One phenomenon he describes is the 'democratic polyphony' of African drumming, where a special kind of empathy is generated in a social group when they play music together (Blacking 1987).

In a very different situation, the crypt of a central London church, I and the other members of the Wednesday Group found much the same musical and social fact. Most Wednesday afternoons for four years up to seven or eight people met in the Marylebone Music Therapy Unit to improvise music together. The initial suggestion for the group had come from the priest in charge of the Counselling Centre within the same building.[1] His idea was both to strengthen the link between the Music Therapy Unit and the Counselling Service and to create a social group around a therapeutic activity. Something was needed, it was felt, to offer clients as well as, or after, one-to-one counselling. His idea also came from the Christian pastoral belief in the power of the group – of people finding both social and spiritual support in meeting together for a creative purpose. The account which follows is not just from my perspective as the therapist, but also includes the comments of the other members of the group. These were taken, with

---

1 The St. Marylebone Centre for Healing and Counselling consisted of three independent but related units – the Music Therapy Unit, the Marylebone Health Centre (a holistic practice with GPs and complementary practitioners), and a drop-in Counselling Centre run by the church.

permission, from two questionnaires I asked people to complete at the end of the first and fourth years of the group.

BEGINNINGS

My idea of a free improvisation group created some initial trepidation. We compromised with a plan of improvising in the first half of the afternoon and listening to music in the second, with a tea-break half way. This arrangement continued for about six months, after which I put the matter to a vote and people opted unanimously to *play* music together rather than listen to it.

The group was designed as a drop-in, open to anyone but with a stable core of 'regulars'. Even more than an individual music therapy session, no group was ever the same. A new person could make both the group and the music quite different, but equally there was also a sense of continuity and development.

The members of the group were also very diverse in age, education and social situation. There was no formal referral structure, people being recommended to try the group by their counsellor or doctor within the Marylebone Centre. Others found the group by a variety of channels. Some had medical, emotional or mental health problems, some were isolated and lonely, some simply wanted to make music with other people. A thought that often struck me during the group was that these widely differing people would not have met in any other situation, and except for the way in which they could create music together there would have been few other ways for them to find a point of contact.

After a shaky start, and a broad learning-curve for all of us, we began to trust in the process of improvising music together. As is often the case in one-to-one music therapy, there were both periods of development and periods of feeling stuck. Then a new person would come into the group, or something less tangible would change, and we would be off again. The group was an experiment for me and for the people who dared to join in. I started off with no explicit theory of group work, and many of the ideas I now have with hindsight come from the comments of members of the group. The account which follows is greatly enriched by what they had to say and I have organised their comments into the categories they seemed naturally to fall. Each of these sections is prefaced with practical descriptions of what happened along with some of my own ideas.

IMPROVISING

We organised the instruments in a rough circle around the grand piano. There was a balance of 'rhythmic' percussion instruments (drums, cymbals, gongs), and melodic ones (xylophone, metalophone, glockenspiel); of large to small instruments.

I gave a simple instruction to the whole group every time a new person joined – that listening was as, if not more important than playing, and that you did not need to play all the time. I also said that we were building the music together – that it was less a chance for 'self-expression' in the way we tend to think of this, but to imagine that the music was almost playing us. I emphasised that everyone there was absolutely necessary to the quality of the music, but no *one* person was, or should feel, individually responsible.

I found that I needed to say less to new people as the group developed. There seemed to be a 'learning curve' in the group as a whole, where the experienced members not only 'taught' the new person to play but, more subtly, taught them to listen. As in one-to-one work in Creative Music Therapy, there were few plans or verbal instructions beforehand. We simply started, whoever was brave enough to make the first sound.

Comments from the group members included:

- We all shared in positioning the instruments, which was somehow less daunting than immediately taking up our posts. I enjoyed the simple directive 'to listen', and felt quite at ease *not* to play as well. Moving around the instruments was fun!
- A roomful of toys and other people to share them with!
- Petrified at first at having to improvise, but soon realised that other people felt the same.
- I felt we're all trying to rediscover some natural, spontaneous element within us...a child-like thing perhaps that enjoys *doing* for its own sake.
- I became more and more fascinated by the freedom and spontaneity.
- To discover that I could spontaneously make music with other people as though we were a jazz quartet was THRILLING. It was deeply fulfilling.
- Sometimes, when I was really flowing, the music seemed to play itself through me. These were the most exciting times for me. Perhaps you might say that my inner musician was allowed out fully to *play*. I could appreciate the thrill that jazz musicians must feel as

they improvise. It is just satisfying in a way complete unto itself. I knew it was good for me by how well I felt afterwards.

CREATING

There was a change in the attitude of the group when people started talking about the improvisations as *their* music, and of it sometimes being beautiful. We usually had time for about three fifteen-minute improvisations, which would mostly come to a natural close. A problem which surfaced quite quickly was the essential passivity of a group of players neither confident with each other or of exactly what they should be doing. I in turn, as the therapist, over-compensated for this by often taking too strong a musical lead and encouraging further passivity.[2] When the group *did* find some confidence, however, a second major problem surfaced – what has been called the 'group beat' – the almost magnetic tendency for the music to get firmly stuck in a single tempo. Understandably it took some time for individual players to dare to initiate a new tempo, rhythm or melodic figure; to change instrument, to stop or start playing. Most of the time I stayed at the piano, not (I hope) from delusions of grandeur, but because I found it the most effective way of 'gluing' the disparate players and the music together. I came to see my role on the piano rather like that of the continuo player in a baroque ensemble – filling in the texture and, when needed, providing impetus and colour.

The sessions were taped, at first just so I could listen back later, as with individual sessions. One week, however, after a particularly beautiful improvisation I suggested we listen back to it. This proved successful, and subsequently we often did this – though not as a ritual and strictly *not* to interpret the music or to criticise the playing. At first the players often commented that they felt they could not 'fit in' to the music and were spoiling it. Hearing it back in a more objective way they found, on the contrary, that they could hardly pick themselves out from the music as a whole.

Comments from the group members included:

- I had to fight the belief that there is a 'right' and a 'wrong' way to do everything and this seemed an enormous opportunity to get it 'wrong'.

---

2 This, of course, is no new problem to any music therapist – it is a central issue of individual music therapy as well. It seemed, however, to be further accentuated by the group situation.

- I learned to shelve the idea of 'this is me about to be creative' – occasionally it just happened without my analysis preceding.
- I see it as a safe place, a sort of laboratory where we can experiment on learning how to give ourselves and each other a good time. The 'innocent' approach – uncluttered by questions of technique, is invaluable. Even if it takes a while to dare to make 'mistakes', it's better to learn from yourself rather than through someone else telling you what to do.
- There was a safe atmosphere in which I (and the others, I think) felt free to experiment and even to 'fail'. There is so little room for attempting and 'failing' – and the space to do that in creative endeavours seems critical to me. 'Fail' is a bad word perhaps, but I mean to say that some things worked better than others, some days went better (musically) than others...but the fact that there was no judgement on the end product – that the focus was on the *process* was such a relief!
- This is the only time in the week I don't feel a failure. Here I feel I'm helping to create something; I feel appreciated.

COMMUNICATING

For many people, living in London is an isolating experience. The counselling unit in the Marylebone Centre also had a 'befriending service' where volunteers would meet a person once a week for a chat. These people did not need professional counselling: their only problem was loneliness. The priest who suggested that I start the group emphasised the social support it could give whilst focusing on some real, creative purpose. Many people came along to the group just to meet people and to have a regular activity to look forward to. Like good English people we incorporated afternoon tea into our timetable, and I always took great care of the purely social aspects of the occasion – how I welcomed people, introduced new people, and so on. But I don't think I deceive myself (from the evidence of the questionnaires) in thinking that there was more to the Wednesday group than 'just' a social occasion. That we were improvising music together added another, different dimension to the quality of communication possible. Many of the people who came to the group were so dramatically different from each other that they had little conventional point of social contact. Yet when we improvised music all the barriers of age, class, education and illness or handicap seemed largely to fall away.

Comments from the group members included:

- Group energy – a sense of heightened energy and *communion* – a very bonding experience.
- When the group changed to match my rhythm or timbre, and looked to me to continue it, I found I would enjoy the prominence for a short while and then rapidly want to fade into the background.
- I love the question and answer effect without words.
- I soon found that I could have a dialogue musically with 'x' that was richer and more interesting than any spoken conversation we'd had. At first we would listen to each other and echo what we heard. As we grew more confident we could respond with variations on the theme – then later adding interesting rhythmic variations and counterpoint. I think we both enjoyed it, and it helped form our friendship. 'X' is a man who otherwise I don't believe I could have got to know, or to like and accept. The music therapy forged the relationship.
- I found it a wonderful forum for exploring musical exchange. It was an opportunity to break down barriers and have some fun!
- I enjoy being creative in the context of a group – and there seems so little of that available in life in any form.
- I always felt closer to the other members of the group afterwards, and had new respect for them.

LISTENING

'Listening is as, if not more, important than playing!' was one of the few instructions I gave the group. From their own experience, however, they also found how to a large extent the quality of the music and the quality of communication between people in the music was dependent on how well they listened. Moreover, there was a sense in which the skill of listening was cultivated over the years by the group as a whole (despite quite large changes of personnel). Once the group was established it seemed to be a quality which could be passed on to new members. Sometimes the reason why a person did not listen was because they came along with a set idea of what a music therapy group was, with the intention of 'expressing themselves'. With others their illness or problem encased them in a bubble of their own activity, preventing them from listening either to themselves or to other people. The other members of the group found it obvious when a person was not listening

– when the loud playing of a single instrument cut across the music. It became increasingly clear to us that good improvisation is as much about good listening as good playing, and that good listening can be heard itself in the playing. You can hear listening, as it were, in the sensitivity of the players' musical response to each other and in their ability to develop a creative idea, to be flexible and yet stable.

We never worked towards making the improvisations beautiful for their own sake, but nevertheless it became increasingly clear that the quality of the music was in direct relation to the quality of the listening. We also discovered that to be listened *to* is the flip-side of listening: that to be listened to is to feel accepted and valued.

Comments from group members included:

- I learned about listening – how important it is to listen to others and how extraordinary it was to be heard by others – exciting, validating, scary! I've learned to communicate by listening to people; to take the initiative, without knowing what will come next.
- I usually found an idea would come by itself, simply by wholly listening to others.
- I gradually learned to widen my field of attention to engage all the members of the group at one time or another.

PLAYING VERSUS SAYING

Many people came to the group surprised both by the lack of instruction and the fact that we did not discuss or interpret the music afterwards. Not interpreting was a conscious policy and no different from how I work with individual clients. Occasionally playing back parts of an improvisation to the group, however, brought an interesting situation. Between the improvisations people would often say things like 'I make such a mess – I can't fit in, I just spoil the music!' But mostly they were pleasantly surprised on hearing the music back on tape to find they *did* fit in (indeed they had usually forgotten which instrument they were playing!). When things went well it was a wonderful feeling to listen back to an improvisation that was effective or beautiful and to feel a sense of pride and achievement together.

An additional rule I made was that when we listened back to a tape we talk only about the qualities of the music itself – what had happened; never who did what or why. This rule was occasionally and happily broken when someone could not help but comment on the beauty or skill of someone else's spontaneous solo. Talking about the 'what?' of the purely musical realm was also part of an indirect training in listening, but still talking was incidental rather than essential.

Another consideration was that there were several people in the group who had less facility with words and concepts than the others. It became obvious to me that whilst the playing included, the words excluded. Moreover, the only moments of conflict in the group in four years happened *outside* the music: in the tea-break or between improvisations. No outright conflict ever happened within the music. I quickly found that the best way of dealing with conflict or averting potential conflict was simply to start playing music together.

Comments from the group members included:

- I have tended to use words as my way into things in the past. I have now learned to trust there are other ways, and music is certainly one of them.
- Not using words was a positive release – there were plenty of smiles and eye contact, often with people I hadn't spoken to before.
- I felt at first as though relating by words would have been much easier, but this soon proved to be wrong. The music flowed more easily than words!
- I was a journalist once – I use words a lot, I have a facility there. It was a relief and a delight *not* to use words, and not to be coming from my head.
- I feel understood here, when I'm playing music, in a way I never feel when I talk to people.

CHANGES

What precedes may suggest everything was too good to be true! In four years of the group there were of course problems, frustrations and times when it simply did not go well. The composition of the group remained roughly constant: an average of six to seven players, a core of regulars attending most weeks for two years or more, supplemented by people who would drop in for a week or two or a longer period. We also had occasional visitors (music therapy students, the odd doctor) who were accepted into the group without fuss, and who helped keep both the social and musical aspects of the group fluid.

There were some of the inevitable problems any group has from time to time, unrelated to it being a music group: of a person being socially or musically dominant; of the group being (very infrequently) intimidating to a new member. Mostly I attempted to deal with such problems indirectly, trusting in the different situation the music gives. This was less the result of any pre-determined strategy and perhaps as much to do with my own personal way of approaching such issues.

The specifically musical problems have mostly been covered earlier – the 'group beat' and habits of playing that included preferred styles and idioms which at worst became repetitive and uncreative. There were also periods when both I as the therapist, and the group as a whole, got into a rut. We had the advantage, however, that the group was not fixed but an ever-varying and open-ended one. A new personality was often enough to give a nudge to a further development, both musically and socially.

As the music therapist I also had difficulties with the group relying on me to lead (or perhaps with myself feeling that I should lead). It took some time for me to work out when to lead, when to leave, when to intervene and when to stand back. I usually kept to the piano, for reasons explained previously – but this meant at times that I unwittingly cultivated excessive dependence on the piano. Again, much of this worked out naturally: the group developed a way of improvising, I developed a way of 'leading'.

One point that came out strongly from all our experience was the fact that skilled listening and musical sensitivity to others had to be balanced against an ability to initiate and take responsibility for the improvisation. Many people made the parallel with their life outside the 'artificial' situation of improvising music together: the problem of remaining open yet confident, sensitive to others yet willing to initiate; being secure yet not dependent; having direction without being dominant; being separate yet together.

Comments from group members included:

- I am a little less inhibited and a little more assertive. I think it is not having any pressure on me to be responsible and perfect. Also I feel part of me is unacceptable, and the improvising makes me feel accepted. Dealing with other people is more difficult but I'm happy I can relate better.
- I always thought of myself as totally incapable of contributing or communicating musically, and it was a delight to find that I could and that music was not just the province of the 'experts'. Empowering personally, and I could see it doing the same for the other members of the group.
- It helped me to realise that even what may seem a fairly insignificant effort on my part can perhaps have a much more significant effect on others than I thought.

- I learned something about my own processes. I saw that sometimes if I found a melody or a pattern that I enjoyed, I liked to stick to it – sometimes getting into a rut. I realise I am wary of change and unadventurous sometimes; and how I behaved musically helped me to see that in a different form.
- No matter how the music went, I always found that whatever mood I'd started in, I felt better after the session.

LISTENING GUIDE

[♫19] The excerpt I have chosen to represent the group comes from a session when five people (including myself) were playing. The instruments used are piano, metalophone, xylophone (both of these pre-set, enabling a G-major/E-minor tonality), conga and a small wooden percussion instrument. The excerpt fades in after the improvisation has been going for approximately two minutes. It shows the improvising of the group at its best – with a sensitive balance of listening, invention and mutual development of the emerging musical material. This was one of those occasions when it felt as if the music was playing us...

CHAPTER 20

Listening

> I learned about listening – how important it is to listen to others, and how extraordinary it was to be heard by others – exciting, validating, scary!

One of the commonest things clients say about their experience of Creative Music Therapy is that they felt listened to – but in a way somehow different than during a spoken conversation. Arguably this chapter on listening should have come first rather than last in a section presenting what happens in Creative Music Therapy. For the real, 'hidden' focus of the approach is about listening rather than playing. In theory as in practice, however, it is usual to see a shift in focus from an initial preoccupation with playing to a recognition of the importance of the kind of listening that develops from a creative musical relationship.

LISTENING AND BEING HEARD

The music therapy group presented in the last case study discovered quite empirically that the quality both of the music they produced and of the feeling of personal contact they had with each other was primarily dependent on one factor – really listening to each other. The epigraph to this chapter is a comment written by a member of that group, and expresses clearly the two aspects of this issue: that the flip-side of being able to listen is the experience of being heard.

Clients in individual music therapy often report similar experiences – of there being a special importance in the kind of listening which can happen through improvisation in music therapy. An unusual example of this happened with a trained musician I worked with, a man I assumed already had a good musical ear (he was trained as a percussionist and had studied composition). In the first five sessions he showed great sensitivity to the sound-world he set about creating for himself with a complex array of instruments. We improvised together as two musicians, though he rejected attempts I made to offer any alternative to the aleotoric and atonal idiom he preferred. My feeling at first was that we played somehow alongside each other rather than together, and only very slowly did any feeling of real musical contact develop. At about this time he said to me at the end of a session, 'I've been wondering what you were going to do with me all this time – as a music therapist that is, rather than just a person to play music with. I've been waiting to see what you do...and now I know what it is – just listening. I feel you hear everything I do...and somehow it feels important.' His comment marked the point from which our work took on a new life – based not on playing differently but on a confidence in each other's intention and ability to listen.

A music therapist is trained to give this quality of listening both to the precise details of the music *and* to the person playing. She listens not to each in isolation but to both together – to the person-in-the-music. In this way the quality of listening she is able to give to the overall musical interaction has both musical and a personal and emotional significance. At the same time, one of the most important benefits the music therapy experience can give to the client is the chance to learn to listen in a new way.

THE ART OF LISTENING

Music has been used by many cultures (both religious and secular) as a training ground for the art of listening (Berendt 1988). Chanting, for example, is a common means of promoting feelings of empathy and social cohesion in groups by having people singing and having to listen carefully to each other as part of a ritual. The first precept of the Benedictine Order – 'Open wide the ears of your heart' – expresses well how the cultivation of listening is not necessarily an end in itself but a means for further emotional, social or spiritual development. Being able to listen implies being open, receptive and sensitive to whatever or whoever addresses us.

In this way listening is more than just hearing. Albeit amazingly complex, the physiology of hearing remains a purely sensory function. Listening, on the other hand, is an intentional act, a skill which can be cultivated. We can only talk of *what* we hear (unless we are an audiologist concerned with the mechanics of hearing), but we can distinguish between different *qualities* (the 'how') of listening. And whilst hearing establishes a subject–object division between you, the hearer, and an aural 'object' out there, listening establishes a relationship *between* things or people, preparing the ground for reciprocal communication (Zuckerkandl 1973).

Ideally (but not always) we both hear and listen to music. Hearing merely registers the fact *that* there is music and where it comes from. Listening, on the other hand, demands a level of sustained concentration but gives a feeling of active involvement and establishes a relationship between you and the music. Background music (whether pop or Mozart) is seldom listened to, and there is a world of difference between how the personal stereo tends to isolate a person in their own world in comparison to the close 'living' listening of the members of an improvisation group, where the music is a focus for intimate communication between them.

For much of the time our specialist Western musical culture allows most people only one form of listening: passively, and for purely aesthetic reasons to someone else's performance. Yet there is another kind of listening that can only come from being an active part of the music-making, what might be called listening-in-playing, or the 'social listening' that is a central focus of many non-Western forms of group music-making. Here it is the social and emotional implications of listening that are paramount. As John Blacking (1987) has commented, what defines a society's real attitude to music is not *what* music they listen to but *how* they listen to it.

LISTENING-IN-PLAYING

This listening-in-playing is central to any musical relationship, be this between a singer and her accompanist, or the members of a string quartet. With improvisation, however, the ability to listen to each other is even more vital to what happens. To people playing music from a score, the eye can still guide the way and keep them on course. Improvisation, on the other hand, is often called 'playing by ear', and its success relies on the imagination of the players and their ability to be acutely sensitive to each others' playing and musical ideas.

Creative Music Therapy is able to use to therapeutic advantage both music's natural cultivation of the art of listening and improvisation's special emphasis on listening-in-playing. Though few people would actually approach a music therapist with the presenting problem of not being able to listen, this can often be a significant accessory to their main problem. The reasons may be quite varied – from the extreme isolation of the autistic child through to people who simply report feeling trapped in the bubble of their own illness, pain or obsession. It is hard for them to be open enough to listen fully and relate to other people and it quickly becomes a vicious circle as they also feel themselves not heard or responded to. People who most need to escape from themselves for a time are often inhibited by the 'noise' of their own mind or body from being able to listen to anything or anyone outside themselves.

Another aspect of the problem is described by Dr Cecil Todes, a psychiatrist who has lived much of his life with Parkinson's disease, and who has experienced Creative Music Therapy. In his book *Shadow over my Brain* he writes, 'There is a complicated interaction in which the Parkinsonian, not being heard is not listened to, so he or she abandons efforts to break through this barrier' (Todes 1990).

Another client told me how she experienced what she called 'getting a resonance' when improvising with me. She was translating from German, and I thought that perhaps she meant 'response'. She said, however, that she did mean 'resonance' in the sense of hearing her own sound sustained as if from a bell. She heard herself being heard, 'I wish life would always be like this – just to get a resonance! What I express in sound this is ME. When someone gives me a resonance, this is communication with *me* – usually what I am I cannot show it.' Is what she describes any different from the 'professional ear' which wise women, priests and psychotherapists have given people in trouble down the years? If there is a difference it lies in the subtly different form of listening possible (and demanded by) a musical relationship. For whilst a spoken dialogue must needs be in alternation, two or more people can play music together at the same time, and can hear an almost simultaneous response or 'resonance' to themselves in the music. In contrast to the priest or the psychotherapist the music therapist typically takes a more continuously active role in improvising music with the client. Yet this involves a fine precision of listening-in-playing, and her listening in turn encourages the reciprocal listening of the client as they respond musically to each other – picking up musical elements, hints of emerging form from each other; echoing, developing and countering them. As the earlier chapter 'Meeting' investigated, it is listening which is the vital condition for making contact in the music and going on to establish the close, creative musical relationship which is at the heart of Creative Music Therapy.

The music therapist's first job, then, is to listen as a *musician* within the session – to be fully conscious and responsive to everything that happens in the purely musical domain. But, at the same time, he also exercises another related form of listening; to the physical and emotional qualities of the client and to how these can be heard in the music or perceived in other ways. Lastly he listens to the quality of the *relationship* between the client and therapist in the music. Being accurate, objective and yet still fully involved in what is happening in the moment during the improvisation is, however, more than most music therapists are humanly capable of. Consequently therapists working in Creative Music Therapy have developed the practice of also listening back to a tape of the session later. This can be a more objective, analytic listening to the tendencies and qualities of the three components: client, therapist and the relationship between them in the music. Nevertheless this 'analytic hearing' is still largely a musical one, concentrating on the purely audible phenomena on the tape. It is foremost a description rather than an explanation of what happened.

FEELING UNDERSTOOD

The music therapist is not always both player and listener. Music therapist Colin Lee's work with Francis, a trained pianist living with AIDS, started off with both of them playing together. After working together for some time the situation changed to Colin often just listening, being a witness to Francis' improvisations. This was still an active listening on the part of the therapist – Francis found he could not play just for himself alone – and it gave the same basic message as a therapist listening *within* playing. It was still an involvement, an understanding shared through the medium of music.

Listening, in most situations, indicates an attempt at understanding. As a client of mine said, 'I feel understood here, when I'm playing music, in a way I never feel when I talk to people.' For some people at least, the experience of listening and of hearing themselves being heard in a musical context seems to be qualitatively different. But equally, as with many other aspects of music therapy, learning to listen differently is not necessarily confined just to the musical process itself, or just to communication between people.

'Listen to your body!' has become one of the slogans of the alternative health movement, and we often use aural metaphors when talking of this kind of awareness. What people call 'inner listening' is really a metaphor for a sensitivity to our whole physical and mental state; it requires the same strategy as listening well to another person speaking, or really listening to music. Good listening is the core of an overall awareness, a mindfullness of our relationship to the whole environment – internal, external, social. Any interference in the quality of listening puts this whole relationship out of balance.

A change of listening is essentially a change of attitude that can influence everything. The whole of this book is about what can happen when dialogue between people is open, responsive and creative. You cannot, however, tell a person to listen differently or better. All you can do is to put them in a situation where a change is necessary and where a different form of listening is demanded and cultivated. In Creative Music Therapy just this happens – an experience of listening differently along with an experience of being heard differently.

Part Three

Understanding the Creative Music Therapy Process

Introduction

Part Two attempted to show some of the main aspects of the Creative Music Therapy process – the musical and personal experiences which can come about because of what is unique in a creative musical relationship.

Questions still remaining may include: what does the client make of these experiences? Does the therapist or the client do anything *with* the material produced in the session (is it verbally interpreted, for example?) If not, what does the client take away from the therapy? Answers to these questions might be expected to help 'qualify' Creative Music Therapy within a traditional understanding of therapy, and to provide areas of investigation to develop a theory or to evaluate the process, its results or even whether it gives value for money.

Part Three tackles some of these questions, beginning with a chapter called 'Reflecting', which looks at the problem music therapy has in fitting into the tradition of therapies where the 'content' of some activity (be this a dream, thought or created image) is verbally reflected upon. It is shown how Creative Music Therapy takes a different view as to the need for there to be anything following the purely musical experience. This is followed by a chapter on evaluation of the music therapy process – a philosophical and methodological problem shared by all the different approaches to music therapy.'Evaluating' examines some of the issues and reviews the recent research completed in the field of Creative Music Therapy.

As in the second part of this book, Part Three interleaves case studies with short essays, and the last two chapters pair a case study of Mathew with a concluding chapter, 'Connecting'. My work with Mathew raised more important questions concerning music therapy (and music) than almost any other. By way of a conclusion the final chapter takes up directly some of these issues, as questions rather than answers. They include: what is the difference between music as experience and music as a form of knowledge? Can and should there be an aesthetics of music therapy? Is musicality a universal underwritten by what Zuckerkandl called 'the facts of the musical experience'? How is music therapy related to musical performance? And lastly, but perhaps most importantly, is music therapy fundamentally a technical 'craft', a means to various relatively defined clinical ends? Or does it remain an artistic activity, and end in itself – with all the potential and capriciousness of any art?

CHAPTER 21

Gisela

Singing means talking from heart to heart
Singing means talking with tone
And eye winking to eye:
Singing gives you legs to stand on the earth.

In the school holidays of her teaching job Gisela admitted herself to the psychiatric ward of the hospital, realising that she needed to find help with the eating disorder and recurrent depression she suffered from. She was an intelligent and attractive woman in her late twenties who had a musical training, played the flute and worked as a music teacher.

In the first session she began to play a drum in a slow tempo, with seemingly disconnected beats. As I joined her on the piano after a while she immediately accelerated into a faster tempo and as I in turn met this she changed to the cymbal. She seemed especially sensitive to any musical contact and tended to withdraw as soon as this occurred.

There appeared to be two almost opposite poles to Gisela's playing: one very controlled but emotionally empty; the other an uncontrolled musical outburst. There seemed little musical ground between the extremes and she had difficulty in any transition. When attempting an accelerando, for example, it became an uncontrolled musical outburst after a certain point, from which she found it hard to escape. My main impression of Gisela's playing was how hard it was for her as a musician to bring to bear some intentional shape on her improvisation.

I suggested she try a melodic instrument and she picked the metalophone and played in the same slow tempo as she had at first on the drum, the

---

Gisela's therapist was Dr Lutz Neugebauer who is joint director of the Institut für Musiktherapie, University of Witten-Herdecke.

melody consisting of only two oscillating tones, expanding eventually to a narrow range of just five, with no noticeable sense of direction or adventure.

In the next few sessions she became more relaxed and I asked her whether she would like to sing. She said she couldn't so I suggested that we could perhaps start by just singing single tones. She agreed to try but found considerable trouble singing even a single tone which she felt fitted the simple accompaniment of open chords I played. She found this upsetting.

In the next session I asked her if she wanted to try singing again. 'Yes, I have to' she said. This, I feared, reflected Gisela's attitude to music therapy in general – that she came more out a sense of duty than enjoyment. Yet at the same time she showed a positive determination to use the opportunity. This time in the improvised singing I was careful not to make her feel isolated or too challenged. I started humming myself to a piano accompaniment which had a clear, repeating harmonic sequence. Gisela joined in and was soon singing fully and expansively, with a confident and beautiful voice. She seemed pleased with herself afterwards. 'I enjoyed it', she said, 'It was good to sing...but it wasn't really me.'

In the next, the seventh session, Gisela came in and said 'today I only want to sing...I won't play because I realise that singing is what's important.' I half expected us to start off in the style of the last session, but Gisela went and sat cross-legged in the middle of the room and began herself. She started to vocalise atonally, then began singing words. I was somewhat perturbed as I heard what she was singing, not just because she had unexpectedly used a text but also because of the immediately emotive and dramatic content: 'I have seen Sodom and Gommorrah, hatred...' she sang, 'I have seen everything...' Had she prepared this before? Should I support it or just listen? My instinct (which I think proved right in retrospect) was to support Gisela *musically*, concentrating on the musical qualities of her 'sprechstimme' rather than getting involved in the obvious symbolic content of the text. There was something new, however, in our playing together apart from the text: a level of contact, invention and the sustaining of one coherent expression and musical mood. This was quite different from anything we had played together before. The spontaneous changes in the improvisation seemed to suggest that, even if the text had been prepared at the beginning, it soon took on an improvised quality. The text of the song is quoted below in full with comments of how the musical aspect changed and reacted to it.

I have seen Sodom and Gomorrah...hatred...I have seen everything with burning eyes.
I've seen torn hearts, I've seen everything and I had to endure it.
Nobody ever said 'Close your eyes', but then I closed them myself.
Nobody ever said 'It's over now – you can open them.'
And when I opened them I was blind...blind and deaf...
I couldn't see any more, I couldn't hear any more.
There was no grief, there was no fury...I was just alone.

[Here there was a musical change: from the dramatic, expressionist style of the opening to a more sustained style]

Only the sun was there
The trees, the animals, the grass – but no people.
Nobody who asks – nobody who listens
Nobody who sees or watches – nobody felt anything...
Everything was hard, as if made of stone: everything was locked up.

[Gisela's voice changed to a child-like tone]

But they *love* you – they've said it.
And you have to be thankful for that.
They've given you nothing, but they want everything:
'But you're our child – be our child!'
I haven't been...and I am not...and I will no longer be...
I've locked them out, and I'll never open the door...to anyone who betrays me...
Who doesn't speak... Speak?... Can be?... Might sing...
Singing means talking from heart to heart
Singing means talking with tone and eye winking to eye
Singing gives you legs to stand on the earth
And who doesn't have legs can't sing, can't walk, can't talk.
Singing means talking from heart to heart.

[The piano depicts the different qualities Gisela sings about]

Warm and soft...jolly or furious...clownish, loud or soft...
Singing means life, singing is truth...
Nobody realises when you sing that you talk from one heart to another,
But some realise (it's sometimes funny!)
If they weren't there I'd be all on my own.
Some realise... It might be that things get better between one person and another...
Can you see me?
Sometimes a tone comes back and brings greetings,
Says 'Good Morning!' and 'We have seen you!'

At this point the words stopped and Gisela and I continued singing for a time without words. The style was by then elegiac, tonal and peaceful. When it came to a stop she said 'that was beautiful' and cried. [20]

I asked Gisela whether she would mind me playing this improvisation to the next case conference on the ward. 'No problem' she said, and talked about the overall musical experience of the session. She seemed genuinely to have forgotten the verbal content of the singing. I emphasised in presenting the work that what was truly remarkable to me was not primarily the content but the musical form: that the improvisation was a long and coherent musical narrative where we shared an equal creative and expressive responsibility. Gisela had dared and succeeded in creating something musically coherent, but not impersonal. She seemed to have found, for the first time in her work in music therapy, a natural balance between her thinking and feeling, and a way of re-finding creativity within her musicianship.

The vocal improvisation was the turning-point in the sessions, which soon had to stop as Gisela went back to her teaching job at the end of the holidays. Shortly afterwards she wrote in a letter to me, 'Music therapy was important to me – it accepted me as I was, and I never felt I had to change. This was what made the changes possible.'

LISTENING GUIDE

[20] Gisela's song (in the original German) is too long to include here complete. Instead the excerpt presents two episodes. The first is the beginning of the song, Gisela beginning in a 'Sprechstimme' style, the therapist accompanying her on the piano, musically echoing her speech rhythms and matching the emotional intensity of her expression in an atonal idiom.

[pause] The excerpt then cuts to a later section of the song, where the musical mood is quite different. Gisela sings: 'Singing gives you legs to stand on the earth, and who doesn't have legs can't sing, can't walk, can't talk. Singing means talking from heart to heart.'

CHAPTER 22

Reflecting

> All the others translate:
> Only your notes are pure contraption,
> Only your song is an absolute gift. (W.H. Auden, *The Composer*)

Two hundred years ago the philosopher Kant wrote about music with some suspicion – remarking that although music obviously affects us, it 'leaves no residue for reflection' (Dahlhaus 1982). It concerned him that music seemed neither to have a 'content' nor to represent something in the way a poem or a painting can. How then do you talk about it? The implications of this problem for music therapy are crucial, since a central aspect of the traditional psychotherapies (and of the arts therapies following in their wake) has been that there is a 'content' of experience or behaviour which can be verbally reflected upon. What happens, then, when musical activity is the central feature of the therapy, given that music seems actively to resist verbalisation? Is it possible to have a therapy (rather than a diverting activity) without a verbal, interpretative element?

'MUSIC THERAPIST'S DILEMMA'

In musicology this problem of talking about music has been dubbed 'Seeger's Dilemma' after the ethnomusicologist Charles Seeger (Cook 1990, Kerman 1985). It concerns how we reconcile what he called 'speech knowledge' which is *about* music (but extrinsic to its process), with 'music knowledge' which is *within* music (and intrinsic to it) – the intuitive and wordless thinking that goes on as part of our playing or listening to music, and which is the locus of the purely musical experience. The difference was nicely illustrated by Chopin who, on being asked by a pupil exactly how to play a difficult etude, said nothing but returned to the piano and played it again, then left the room.

'Music Therapist's Dilemma' I would suggest is even more acute. Most music therapists, of whatever tradition or training, are using for the great part of the work their 'music knowledge' as musicians when they play music with clients. But they also need to talk about their work – and it is the music the client or the client and therapist have played which is the main object of that reflection. One of the main differences in approach to music therapy lies in whether or not the therapist uses the music as material for verbal reflection within the session with the client, and how this is done. A previous section in Chapter 4 showed how some music therapy currently practised is best characterised as 'music psychotherapy', where the music played *is* used as an object of subsequent reflection between client and therapist, and where the musical element is only part of a broader conception of therapy. The additional theory (which must operate in the form of 'speech knowledge') becomes both a method of working in the session, and a way of explaining the process as a whole. In this way music therapy is subsumed within something else – mostly psychodynamic theory. The issue then becomes not just a problem of talking about music, but of *how* this is done – the matter of interpretation. Here Kant's dilemma has in a way been solved – the therapist has found her 'residue for reflection', but at the same time many thorny issues for music therapy have been raised.

MUSIC AND WORDS

As mentioned before, Freud's attitude to art and creativity was decidedly ambiguous. What was less ambiguous was his aversion to music, which in the words of his nephew Harry, he 'despised' (Storr 1992). A consequence of this is that both Freud's theories, and those of the other founding fathers of psychoanalysis, have almost nothing to say about the nature and function of music. This omission is perhaps explained not only by a personal aversion to music, but also by a more theoretical issue. For, unlike the worlds of both words and visual images, music steadily resists the process of excavation and verbalisation of symbolic meanings and ambiguities – the very process that the psychoanalytical principle is based on. That, in short, talking about music is difficult.

In contrast to Freud, Jung liked his patients to paint or write for themselves as part of their analysis, and he was evidently enthusiastic about an early development of music therapy he came across (Hitchcock 1987). But he also wrote, in *The Practice of Psychotherapy*, 'The mere execution of the pictures is not enough. Over and above that an intellectual and emotional understanding is needed; they require to be not only rationally integrated with the conscious mind, but morally assimilated' (Jung 1954). In other words, the experience of the art-form is not enough in itself: something has to be done with it. Indeed I think this would be a common image of therapy – that something is made of what the client says or does; that psychotherapy is not just talking, or the arts therapies just painting or just playing music. This 'something' which is done over and above is a process of reflecting verbally on the experience and its possible meanings within the inner and social life of the client. Jung called psychotherapy a 'spagyric art', meaning a two-fold process which aims to start with an analysis and end with a new synthesis of the client's personality (Stevens 1991). He saw art as a useful catalyst to both processes, but only when 'rationally integrated' by talking about it within an already prescribed scheme of interpretation. But here we are back with 'Music Therapist's Dilemma': how we can reconcile the musical process (thinking *within* music) in any meaningful way with thinking and talking *about* music – especially when it is not a musicologist talking about the work of a dead composer but a music therapist of the improvisation of a living person who has come for help.

Jung's 'rational integration', or any other process of interpretation, reflection or 'verbal processing' must use words, and the process must work in the way language works. In contrast the main argument of this book has been that essentially music therapy works in the way music works. This point involves no critique of psychotherapy or psychodynamic theory *per se*, but an attempt to demonstrate that the basic difference between how music and words work has basic implications for any music therapy.

Zuckerkandl (1973) is clear in his distinction between what he calls 'musical thought' and 'logical thought' and their respective functions. Whilst the latter involves words, concepts and propositions, 'musical thought' is essentially productive and creative, 'it deals with motions and links them into patterns:

> Logical thinking is deductive, brings something to light, its goal is to discover the hidden; it is like developing an exposed photographic plate... Musical thinking articulates, gives form to an amorphous impulse; its goal is to fulfil; it is like the development of a living being, self-development. (Zuckerkandl 1973)

Psychotherapy is at base a form of 'logical thinking' (in Zuckerkandl's sense); operating through words and working the way words work – to divide subject from object, to analyse, to question. Any use of psychotherapeutic techniques within music therapy must also work this way. The music (whether improvised or heard receptively) must become an object of examination, for both therapist and client *after* the experience of playing or hearing it. To do this several assumptions have to be made about music. First, that is has a 'content' (that it can be *about* something) and second, that it can be symbolic (it can stand for something else). In psychodynamic theory the process of asking 'What does it mean?' is called interpretation – in the words of psychoanalyst Peter Lomas (1987) 'the process of relating two different sets of things, or of converting one set of things into another'. Interpretation is also central to many critical responses to art: 'a conscious act of the mind which illustrates a certain code, certain "rules" of interpretation' (Sontag 1966).

> Directed to art, interpretation means plucking a set of elements (the X, the Y, the Z, and so forth) from the whole work. The task of interpretation is virtually one of translation. The intepreter says, Look, don't you see that X is really – or, really means – A? That Y is really B? That Z is really C? (Sontag 1966)

Any interpretative system needs a guiding theory, and the problem with a psychoanalytical interpretation of music or music in therapy is that this basic theory is missing as regards the key phenomenon under question – music. Hence a lot of ideas must be borrowed from other areas.

An approach to music therapy developed from the mainline psychoanalytic tradition is 'Analytical Music Therapy'. I want to present this in some detail in the next section in order to juxtapose the differences and similarities between this understanding and that of Creative Music Therapy.

AN EXAMPLE OF AN INTERPRETATIVE MUSIC THERAPY: 'ANALYTICAL MUSIC THERAPY'

'Analytical Music Therapy' was developed by Mary Priestley, who defines her approach as 'The symbolic use of improvised music by the therapist and client to explore the client's inner life and provide the proclivity for growth' (Priestley 1983).

Here the attitude is unashamedly that the purely musical element can and should be talked about and that the improvisations are representations of thoughts, feelings and images from the client's inner world. Instructions are often given about the improvisation to follow and interpretations made afterwards. The intention is that the purely musical experience be used therapeutically. In an article in the *Journal of British Music Therapy* called 'Music and the Listeners' Mary Priestley (1988) describes her work with a client who was herself a psychotherapist and who came to music therapy with the specific problem of not being able to play the piano in front of other people without considerable anxiety. Hours of verbal therapy had failed to help the problem. After discussing how music related to her past, Priestley asked the woman 'to play in the role of the "The Listeners", hoping that she might get back her projections of her punitive and self-critical parts'.[1] After the improvisation they discussed it. The therapist describes the character of another improvisation, called 'Stealing Father': 'She played grasping, grabbing, triumphant music to my drum and cymbal.' She then says to the client, 'I said the music represented a very intimate phantasy relationship with her father that went way back and that it explained the guilt when she was discovered playing. She agreed.' Mary Priestley has developed various techniques of improvisation which extend this way of working. As therapist she will sometimes take a non-playing role such as 'super-ego' against the client's playing. Improvisations or sessions are linked with the logic of the images, thoughts and interpretations which come up in the verbal processing of the playing. A short dialogue is included in 'Music and the Listeners' from the therapist's notes about the end of the third session, when the client cried, 'She wept. I asked if she cried because she felt understood. "No. Just responded to."'

The case has an interesting conclusion, where both therapist and client (looking back several years to the work) write about the sessions. The therapist concludes that:

> The sessions gradually uncovered the client's association of music with her intimate phantasy relationship with her father, but because this knowledge was not enough without repeated reality-testing in the present, the session continued until her playing and improvising became freer and more enjoyable.

The client, on the other hand, remembers the work as good, but nothing of the verbal aspects, the interpretations.[2] What she does remember and consider significant about the sessions was, 'I also loved making music with someone. Memorable moments were when I discovered I could sing, and that, to me, my voice sounded clear and an important and integral part of the ensemble of percussion and piano.'

---

1 All subsequent quotations are from the 1988 article.

2 I am aware, however, that therapists working in a psychodynamic way would in any case consider this normal.

'MUSIC PSYCHOTHERAPY' IN RELATION TO CREATIVE MUSIC THERAPY

It would be fair to add, however, that not all music therapists who use a combination of playing and talking within their sessions would be working to as rigorous a psychoanalytic credo as Mary Priestley. Psychodynamic theory has developed since Freud, and music therapists have likewise included some later models, such as 'object-relations theory' and the related observational work of mother–infant non-verbal communication into their own clinical model of music therapy (Bunt 1994). More recent terms such as 'music psychotherapy' and 'psychodynamically informed music therapy' have attempted to soften the boundaries between music therapy and psychotherapy.[3]

Though perhaps representing increasing diversity, both 'music psychotherapy' and 'psychodynamically informed music therapy' nevertheless define themselves in reference to classic psychoanalytic principles and conventions. To a certain extent, of course, almost any therapy borrows from these: the conventions of confidentiality, reliability and the relative consistence of the time and place of the sessions being the most obvious. When music therapy is subsumed within a psychodynamic approach, however, there are also a set of underlying theoretical assumptions which are more than simply conventions of the therapeutic context. These are, in short, that:

1. Music is a bridge between unconscious and conscious process.
2. Music is a symbolic phenomenon and can, within the music therapy situation, express or represent something that can be interpreted and articulated in words.
3. Music facilitates the development of words.
4. Verbalisation, indicative of a bringing to consciousness, is necessary to the therapeutic process.
5. The 'dynamic relationship' between therapist and client is a necessary focus of the therapeutic process and consequently also needs to be an object for examination, interpretation and verbal processing.

---

3 David John's (1992) article 'Towards Music Psychotherapy' tackles these issues. A further discussion section in the same issue of the *Journal of British Music Therapy* concerns the relationship between music therapy and psychotherapy and gives a cross-section of current views on the subject.

This stance is conveniently summed up in David John's statement, 'This process of music being literally a medium through which unconscious material can bypass repression and become conscious in words forms the basis of music psychotherapy' (John 1992). For the time being I leave it to the reader to contrast this stance with that taken by the therapists who have presented their work in the present book.

A third possible position in the relationship between music therapy and psychotherapy might be that of the many music therapists who would argue that there should be no firm boundary between words and music; that the therapist should notice and work with *any* elements which carry an expressive function – a client's gestures or the 'music in the speech'. Working 'only on the notes' is a limitation and a constriction in this view. Equally they may argue that, though they do not believe psychodynamic theory to be an explanation of the music therapy process overall, it *can* offer a useful model in helping understand many things that happen within the therapy situation – issues of relationship, power, dependence, and so on.

Music therapists working within the tradition of Creative Music Therapy may agree with much of this, and may well need all the help available in trying to understand the variety of potentially difficult situations their work can bring. Additionally, few therapists working to a 'mostly musical' model do not speak to their clients, discuss what is happening sometimes, and deal if necessary with what is 'extra-musical'. The central issue is that whilst psychodynamic theory may well be one useful way of understanding the nature and problems of the therapeutic *situation*, it is not an adequate explanation of the central, transformative locus of that situation – the music-therapeutic *process*. And it is this which Creative Music Therapy attempts to understand, refine and make accessible to people.

UNDERSTANDING OR RESPONSE?

The issue in this chapter concerns what our clients get *essentially* from the experience of music therapy. Whether it is some new knowledge, insight, understanding; or a mostly wordless, concept-less experience which is first and foremost a musical one. The former can only come through what Zuckerkandl (1973) called 'logical thought' whereas the latter, an experience resulting from 'musical thought', is the natural result of music-making in any context.

If, in Creative Music Therapy, the therapist is not making interpretations or obviously doing anything with the 'content' of the music and the session, then what *is* he or she doing? We are back to the now familiar question: 'Are we *just* making music with people?'. A start to an answer lies perhaps in the reply Mary Priestley's client gave when asked whether she cried because she felt 'understood'. 'No,' she said, 'just responded to.' When we talk about music rather than words, 'understanding' seems the wrong term. Stravinsky, when asked if he understood some piece, said, 'I haven't understood a bar of music in my life – but I've *felt* it!' This is perhaps nearer to the central message that comes out of the case studies in this book and from the comments of the clients: that they did not necessarily find new insights, knowledge or advice which could be stated propositionally – not all the things that words and 'logical thought' can provide. Rather, they found a very different *experience* of themselves – one in contrast to the usual physical and emotional patterns dictated by pathology or habit. This experience was a direct result of how music and a creative musical relationship works.

A MUSICAL INTERPRETATION

It is, however, possible to talk both of musical 'understanding' and 'interpretation' when this is something happening purely *within* the process of making music or listening to it. A pianist or a conductor are said to be 'interpreters' of a musical score – they convert the notes on the page into a performance which makes sense of the music. This is certainly a process of understanding but certainly *not* one of explanation where you can ask in words '*what* do you understand?' This is perhaps why performers can seldom explain exactly *why* they do what they do – the logic is intrinsic to the whole process, where an interpretation is a creative response to the piece in the time of its performance. The literary critic George Steiner writes of this:

> Interpretative response under pressure of enactment I shall, using a dated word, call 'answerability'. The authentic experience of understanding – when we are spoken to by another human being or a poem, is one of responding responsibility... We are answerable to a text, to the work of art, to the musical offering in a very specific sense, at once moral, spiritual and psychological... Responsible response, answering answerability make of the problem of understanding a moral act. (Steiner 1989)

I want to suggest that this is essentially no different from what a therapist does in Creative Music Therapy in the time of the improvisation with the client – that this is the locus of what happens in, and what is essential to, the therapeutic process. As one of the members of the music therapy group said, 'I feel understood here when we're playing music together, in a way I never feel when I'm communicating with words.'

But what exactly is this form of understanding? I will (experimentally) call it '*intrinsic* interpretation' in contrast to the *'extrinsic'* psychodynamic method which makes symbolic translations of one thing into another (for example, Mary Priestley's statement that 'the music represented a very intimate phantasy relationship with her father'). In contrast the 'intrinsic interpretation' of the music therapist is itself a musical response *within* his playing with the client; it is a 'musical understanding' of the playing of the client – a creative response to the overall musical fabric which is the 'musical between' that includes both the client and the therapist in the music.

All of this can be seen in microcosm in the example in the earlier chapter, 'Just a Minute...'. Here the therapist's response within the music is not just an accompaniment or a passive echoing of the client's playing but an active response, a creative 'interpretation' of it: working to encourage, imitate, explore, extend, give a context to, sometimes check, the playing of the client. In this case her playing was at first tentative and unformed and needed an appropriate 'interpretative response'. In a different case the client may be playing in the opposite way – loud, continuous music which seems stuck, uncreative and unresponsive to a musical relationship between client and therapist. Here the therapist's 'intrinsic interpretation' will attempt to work the other way – to pose musical contrast, encourage changes in speed and dynamics, and a recognition of how both players can share the responsibility for the music. In this way it is clear that this 'interpretative response' can also be at the same time a clinically directed *intervention* – an intentional decision by the therapist that a certain musical direction is needed at that moment. There is, then, a simultaneity within this process: of the therapist's perception of what is happening musically; of an 'interpretative response' to the client in the music; of a level of musical intervention as necessary; of the mutual response to the creative possibilities of the music as a whole. None of this is verbalised or even necessarily conceptualised outside the time of the music itself. Instead it is the second-by-second realisation of what I characterised in Part Two of this book as the main experiences of Creative Music Therapy: meeting, creating, expressing, recalling, listening... At each stage the therapist hears, responds, answers; the client experiences being heard, being responded to, being answered.

CONCLUSION

In the previous case study the verbal content of Gisela's song could be seen in a number of ways: as literal and autobiographical, as imaginative and symbolic, as simply creative. The therapist, however, did not work with the verbal content of the song outside of the time of the music but supported and responded to it creatively but specifically musically – echoing the speech rhythms of her 'Sprechstimme', helping give continuity and form to the 'surface' of her expression. What seemed significant for Gisela in this breakthrough session was not *what* she had begun singing (she had forgotten this a week later), but the nature of the purely musical experience: that she had sustained a long and coherent musical narrative; that she had shared equal creative responsibility for it with the therapist; and that, quite simply, she had created something beautiful.

In *Against Interpretation* Susan Sontag writes:

> Our task is not to find the maximum amount of content in a work of art, much less to squeeze more content out of the work than is already there. Our task is to cut back content so that we can see the thing at all.
>
> The aim of all commentary on art now should be to make works of art – and, by analogy, our own experience – more, rather than less, real to us. The function of criticism should be to show *how it is what it is*, even *that it is what it is*, rather than to show *what it means*. (Sontag 1966)

Because the common expectation of the therapeutic process is one of reflecting *on* something (a meaning, an action, etc.), it seems that this does not fit what happens essentially in the process of Creative Music Therapy. Perhaps a change of metaphor is needed. The visual term 'reflect' indicates the use of words and logical thought to stand back as a subject observing an object. 'Extrinsic interpretation' then relates this to something else – says 'In other words...'. On the other hand, what happens in music and music therapy would perhaps be better described by the aural metaphor of 'resonance'. The non-verbal, non-conceptual experience comes as a resonance *within* the music, where there is often not the usual separation between the music as the object with the players as subjects (Ansdell 1990).

This idea of the musical 'resonance' is one of the central defining factors people have continually returned to as a feature of the musical experience. Consequently, what the therapist does within the music therapy situation in Creative Music Therapy – the process I have characterised in this chapter as 'intrinsic interpretation' – is not the 'putting in other words' of verbal logic but a metamorphic process which says 'the same but different' – a helping in articulating the constant change and growth of given material which is the hallmark of musical thought and musical communication. With this I think we are nearer to an approach to, and an explanation of, music therapy which is more consistent with what happens in music as a whole.

CHAPTER 23

Jane

> A few days after the sessions I had an interesting dream: me, standing at the centre of the universe – quite alone, but not lonely. I heard myself singing, wonderful tunes – I almost couldn't believe it. And I heard myself singing to the world: 'I can sing again.'

This case study presents an attempt at finding methods of researching the process of Creative Music Therapy. It was unusual within this tradition in that it involved an equal collaboration between three people – the client, a music therapist and a researcher (Jane, Rachel Verney and David Aldridge respectively). This account makes use of the viewpoint of each of these three, showing both the process and the problems of such a study.

David Aldridge: Our basic questions were, is it possible to find a method for examining the process of Creative Music Therapy without just taking on board another theoretical model? and second, how do people talk about the *experience* of music therapy? We wanted to start making use of the comments and insights of those adult clients who were able to articulate something of their experience. It was therefore helpful that, as a musician, Jane already had a musical vocabulary with which she could begin to describe her experiences in music therapy.

The project was also an experiment to see whether the work could remain genuine therapy whilst also being investigated. The idea was that I should

---

Rachel Verney trained as a music therapist with Paul Nordoff and Clive Robbins. She worked as a music therapist in Germany and Denmark, at the Nordoff-Robbins Music Therapy Centre in London and subsequently set up the Marylebone Music Therapy Unit in central London in 1985. Dr David Aldridge has been involved in developing appropriate strategies to research Creative Music Therapy since 1987. He is professor of clinical methodology at the Universität Witten-Herdecke, Germany.

actually be in the therapy room as an observer whilst the therapy took place. This was an attempt to reconcile two notions: first, that an observer cannot totally understand a process like Creative Music Therapy without being (be it passively) part of it; but that, second, that if he *is* there he is influencing it and therefore cannot have an objective view of it. These questions were themselves part of the investigation.

The aim was to collect data from several view points about a short-term course of therapy. Jane was asked to keep a diary of the process which she wrote after every session. She was encouraged to express her thoughts and feelings in the diary in any way she felt appropriate (though these were never verbally discussed in the music therapy sessions). A second view point came from the music therapist, who also used the tapes of the sessions. As an additional observer I built up a perspective from which to understand the descriptions of the therapist and client – an observer of observations, as it were.

The only preparations were that I got to know Jane briefly before the sessions and agreed to leave the session if either the client or therapist requested.

Rachel Verney: 'What I want to find out is whether the problem with my hand is organic or psychological?' Jane told me. In her late thirties, she was an articulate and somewhat earnest woman who was a trained musician, playing and teaching the flute for a living. The problem with her hand, for which she seemed to be able to find no answer, had limited her playing in the last few years. She had come across music therapy through a friend who was a music therapist, and had heard a talk I had given. Consequently, Jane came to her own sessions knowing what it would entail and with a sense of commitment. Owing to circumstances the only way we were able to work together was to have a one-off intensive week of sessions: one per day for five days. My part of the bargain was to ask Jane if she would agree to collaborate with the research project. She was happy to do so.

During the five days she did nothing other than the music therapy sessions. This arrangement was unusual, and it was certainly a question for me whether it would be at all satisfactory – or whether the more usual weekly gap between sessions was necessary to assimilate the experience. The account which follows of our five sessions together comes from my own notes and from Jane's diary.

Session 1: Standing in front of a drum and cymbal Jane played with determination. She made lots of stops and starts and could not seem to find any flow in the music. It also had little playfulness: every musical action seemed thought out and controlled and with an insistent 'dead beat'. It didn't sound like the playing of someone I knew was musically trained and could play the flute well.

What is interesting, however, is the discrepancy between my initial perceptions and Jane's experience:

> **Jane session 1:** Musical relationship develops. Very soon felt that what I expressed was being understood. Feel accepted.
>
> Second improvisation (2 drums, 2 cymbals, 2 sticks): Wider possibilities of sound quality give a feeling of freedom, like a bird in a cage having the door opened. I enjoy 'flying', making real music, feel my heart. The instruments sing in my soul; I get very warm; my breath flows, is wide. I completely forget David is in the room.

Strangely, there was little singing quality when Jane played a melodic instrument (the xylophone), and when she actually sang it seemed constricted and unmelodic, with little sense of phrasing. She wrote herself 'It's not easy for me – ambivalence of feeling well and in prison. I feel weak, no power all over.' After the first session I had quite clearly in my mind what might be possible in the following sessions with Jane. She herself concluded after the first day: 'I lived very deep in the music. Rachel and I gave and took.'

Session 2: In the improvisations I confronted Jane's musical 'safety': the controlled, organised playing that seemed to take no risk or to have any playfulness. She begins her diary entry for the second session by saying 'the atmosphere of the room depresses me – I remember my school', and later,'I meet myself.'

In the first improvisations where she played drums and cymbals my music on the piano posed direct contrasts: jagged discords and irregular rhythms against her neat regularities; syncopations against her insistent pulse; teasing playfulness against her earnestness. I was being musically provocative and challenging. She reacted but never responded in kind. She seemed lost, had no response to make to this situation. In moments she found the strength to chance less order, but even her attempt at chaos was relatively ordered. Jane writes about this session in what, at first, sounds like euphemism, 'A lot of music and I enjoyed it enormously. There is very close communication between me and Rachel. I feel completely alive in the music...but my hands, feet and whole body felt cold.' There was in a sense this coldness in her attempt to play melody or sing. Her playing of the xylophone was defined by its rhythm rather than melody, and her voice strained, the melody uncontrolled. It seemed almost unnatural for her. Jane writes: 'Singing – feel very stressed, hardly possible though I do it... I feel the policeman in my neck, the old Jane problem.' I too felt exhausted by the session.

Session 3: Jane arranged the instruments and her chair so that her back was to me. Rather than being a hostile gesture this emphasised the closeness in the purely musical relationship made solely through listening. She comments, 'with my back against the piano – the possibility of listening differently to the music. Communication with Rachel very intensive.'

Jane began to dare more, made more initiatives, took more risks. We played an atonal improvisation which encouraged these qualities, 'Atonal improvisation without fixed rhythm absolutely detonates the gates and leads to a kind of "micro" and "macrocosmos" of musical expression... At last deliverance from fixed patterns. That's what I was longing for.'

Session 4: Jane sang for most of the session on the fourth day. It was hard for her; the strain came out in the quality of the voice, which sounded forced but also vulnerable. She tried hard, too hard, and her vocal melody sounded controlled and pedantic rather than the flying she seemed to long for. Jane wrote, 'I felt "spastic" in my voice and pelvis – my voice doesn't grow.'

I worked on specific ways in this session to help Jane to feel more involved and at ease with her voice: getting her to sing single tones related to her natural breath, then expanding out the voice into melody, almost for the first time by herself. The improvisation developed into a duet between us – a slow melody in E major with our voices weaving in and out of each other. As we sang her voice seemed to warm up.[ɷ21] At the end of the session I suggested we sing a scherzo and we managed a wonderful two-minute miniature of unaccompanied singing – a comical, atonal burst of shrieking which left us both laughing.[ɷ22] She had finally showed real playfulness and invention, using her voice in quite a different way, with life and spirit. She wrote herself, 'Legato singing is possible as I imagine myself playing the flute. The first time David disturbs...singing is so intimate! The atonal singing wonderful...Rachel got me! Altogether a good feeling after this session.'

Session 5: Even more so than the previous session Jane was *involved* with her voice, involved in her music in the improvisations. Her singing had a sense of melody and direction, and also space and breath. But where she really sang was in her playing, especially in a piano duet we played towards the end. It was a breakthrough not just in its melody and simplicity, but also in the feeling that this was the most authentic and honest music we had made in these sessions. Instead of being ordered and forced, finally the music felt pulsed and breathed and sang:

> Improvisation on the piano – great joy! I can hardly believe it's possible for me. Starting with one finger, one tone, I let it grow, and afterwards playing with both hands. With Rachel so much more music-making comes by itself... It's possible to *sing* on the piano. I felt that each tone under my fingers was living, not just mechanical.

For me as the therapist the work in a single week was hard – almost too hard. I had the feeling that much the same process would have happened if we had worked more conventionally over a six-week period. The practical restrictions on both of us made this impossible, and it was interesting for me to see that the musical work within music therapy has a progression, almost like music itself, which has its own space and time.

David Aldridge: Jane came to music therapy with the 'presenting problem' of her wrist, and a question to the music therapist as to whether the therapy might be able to show her whether the problem was physical or psychosomatic. Within the 'medical model' an evaluation of music therapy might in this case rest at its simplest level on symptomatic relief – whether the wrist improved, or, at a slightly more subtle level, on whether Jane found out something about the nature of her problem.

However, in her own account of what was important to her about the music therapy the problem with her wrist does not even feature. Rather than being questioned on 'before' and 'after' effects Jane was left free to express in any way she felt appropriate how she had experienced the process of the music therapy. She did this mostly through her diary entries, which included both musical description using musical terminology and also emotionally expressive comments about her feelings in the situation. She supplemented this with a letter she sent me later, summing up her experience of the sessions:

> The intensive work, the self-confrontation in the music therapy was very, very exhausting. My whole body felt heavy at times. But out of this exhaustion and heaviness grew a very new power, physically and emotionally... In this concentration music therapy felt like looking in a mirror, facing oneself. I experienced that all the possibilities in music – if they are used creatively and sent into the centre of us – are like a self-regulating system. My singing, my making music has really changed, and also the way I listen has changed. Also I realised that it doesn't matter if one, two or three therapists are in the room – it's possible to be totally involved in the whole process and not be distracted.

> A few days after I had worked with Rachel I had an interesting dream: me standing at the centre of the universe, quite alone (yet not lonely) and I heard myself singing, wonderful tunes, I almost couldn't believe it. And I heard myself saying to the world: 'I can sing again, I can sing again.' My voice sang out into the distance. This was the culmination for me...my singing...

Jane chose to express what was most important to her about the music therapy sessions by writing about a dream – albeit a dream about a musical experience.

When talking about single-case studies as a way of researching music therapy I often use this work as an example of what we should be prepared to include in any investigation into music therapy. To Jane it seemed that the dream was as important as the fact of any medical improvement of the wrist. If we throw away the dream we throw away what is important to the whole thing. We also impoverish science by ignoring such phenomena.

This work was partly a study into the possibility of making a study, and as such showed the potential of the single case to yield varying data over time in differing discourses, and how this data can serve to orientate further useful questions. One point that came out of the study was that we cannot expect a standardised reaction from clients – we have to respect and be able to use the different ways people choose to express their thoughts and feelings about an experience – using whatever language is available to them. By having, in this study, three observational viewpoints we could begin to examine both the commonalities and the differences in how people talk about an experience of music therapy.

We also demonstrated that a professional observer is mildly disturbing though not necessarily destructive to the process – and that it remained therapy under investigation rather than becoming an artificial experiment. This itself may have something to do with the nature of the relationship between client, therapist and music in Creative Music Therapy – a matter itself for possible future investigation.

LISTENING GUIDE

[21] Jane stands next to the piano, looking serious. This excerpt fades into Jane singing alone, accompanied by the therapist on the piano. Her voice is in a high register, sounding strained – as if she is uncomfortable singing. The therapist provides her with a warm harmonic support and, when Jane's voice becomes lower in register, the therapist joins her and the improvisation becomes a duet. The music is warm and expansive, with a more shaped phrasing developing naturally from the breathing of the two singers. Jane beomes totally concentrated, confident and involved in the music.

[♒22] Jane stands next to the piano, relaxed and full of vitality. She sings an atonal, upturned phrase which the therapist answers with a mock-intense vibrato, their voices sliding and shrieking over a wide range of pitches. They both enjoy the energy, drama and freedom of this improvisation, suddenly landing together at the end, bursting into laughter...

CHAPTER 24

Evaluating

> Research must be held accountable for the choice of its rationality. (Michel Foucault)

QUESTIONS OF ART: QUESTIONS OF SCIENCE

'Is there proof that it works?' is perhaps inevitably the most difficult of the difficult questions you get asked as a music therapist. How this question is intended will to an extent depend on the setting in which the music therapist works, and what the dominant school of thought is there. This may range from a largely educational model in a special school through to a psychodynamic one in a therapeutic community or the 'medical model' of a hospital or clinic.

Consequently, questions concerning evaluation of the effects of music therapy are often difficult to answer satisfactorily, not because of lack of information or experience, but because of the form and preconceptions of the questions. These point to the somewhat precarious tightrope the music therapist finds him or herself on – with on the one side art, subjectivity and issues of quality, and on the other the focus on quantity and objectivity, and a tradition of research methodologies originating in natural science. Most of all, as research in the field has begun to find its feet in the last ten years, music therapist researchers have had to be careful to ensure that what they believe to be the central components of their work do not disappear under the microscope of traditional research methodologies. It is yet another aspect of the tightrope – keeping to the 'big questions' and not slipping into studying, in Roger Bannister's phrase 'either the vaguely significant or the specifically irrelevant' (Reason and Rowan 1981).

Given that this book is not intended to be a survey of the whole of current music therapy, neither does the present chapter attempt to review all current research. I merely want to look at some of the issues involved in evaluating and researching the approach being presented here – Creative Music Therapy.[1]

LOOKING IN THE RIGHT PLACE

'Music therapy is coming of age but there is still a need to demonstrate efficacy', writes Leslie Bunt (1994). Most music therapists, however, feel no need to give 'hard proof' of the value and effectiveness of their work. They choose to present not statistical, but directly observable evidence of its worth and appropriateness – playing tapes and showing videos of the work in action, backed up with an explanation of the basic principles. It has been the argument of this book that in Creative Music Therapy there is no hidden agenda which qualifies it as 'therapy' and that the fundamental experience is simple and readily understandable and observable in its own terms – the benefits of a creative musical communication within a sustained, dependable relationship. Indeed most of the questions people typically ask about Creative Music Therapy are not requests for proof but more practical ones, such as a parent or doctor asking, would music therapy be suitable for an autistic child? or, in what way is music therapy suitable for an adult with cancer? These can be answered primarily from the music therapist's experience and own evaluation of the process for different people and problems.

Another level of enquiry cannot, however, be answered so casually. As the music therapy profession has become more established so too has an expectation for a more critical examination of its processes and of the effectiveness of its interventions. Published research studies may give a doctor confidence to refer patients, and a manager of therapeutic services in a health authority may have to make financial and political decisions on the basis of such evidence. Both may make the perhaps doubtful claim that most other treatments (be they pharmaceutical or rehabilitatory) have undergone some form of objective scrutiny into both their method and outcome. And do not patients have the right to enquire critically about the service they may be paying for? Certain aspects of this argument are, of course, fair – but lead to an essentially false comparison. A new drug certainly needs the rigour of quantitatively based trials which conform to the basic norms of medical science: relative objectivity, generalisability, repeatability and reliability. In-

---

1 Much of course can be learned from the research work of both music therapists working within other approaches and from the research work of other arts therapists – all of whom face similar problems. See Gilroy and Lee (1995) and Payne (1993).

vestigation into the art therapies, however, needs quite different parameters: for, as E.M. Forster commented, 'the arts are not drugs' and their central creative component is both 'mysterious and capricious'(Sacks 1991). These characteristics are alas not very suited to the traditional research methodologies. Most of the important aspects of the music therapy process are neither predictable, generalisable, objectively verifiable or even reliable. Most of all they are not *quantifiable* in any way – the basic experiences of contact, creativity, form and beauty cannot be accommodated within research which starts with quantitative questions of 'How much…?'

Additionally, music therapy is a highly individual pursuit on all levels. Within the very basic parameter of using improvised music as the basis of a therapeutic relationship, almost every other variable is individual: the strategy and music of the therapist; the problems and abilities of the client; what actually happens in each improvised (and therefore by definition unpredictable) session. If what is vital to the situation is essentially variable then this sits very uneasily with any quantitative attempts to iron out just this aspect with the generalisation of statistical control and the randomisation of clients in classically designed clinical trials.[2]

Kenneth Aigen sounds a further necessary warning: that, in researching music therapy, we should take care not to reify the profession itself. It is possible that this will make us look in the wrong place:

> Gaining a true understanding of the personal transformation characteristic of therapeutic growth necessitates that our explanatory efforts go beyond categories like client, therapist, health, illness and clinical intent. These elements are the supportive social edifice that allow and enable the transformative process to occur, but they do not provide the impetus upon which the process turns… In our research efforts we have made the mistake of attributing explanatory significance to the components of the *profession* of music therapy – the realm that we define through convention – rather than looking to the elements of the *discipline*…[which] lie buried and await discovery in the intuitions, actions and tacit knowledge of our most gifted music therapists. (Aigen 1991)

---

2 For references on music therapy in the medical literature see: David Aldridge (1993a), 'Music Therapy Research I: A Review of the Medical Research Literature within a General Context of Music Therapy Research'.

DEVELOPING MUSIC THERAPY RESEARCH

Given all the problems that seem to be inherent in investigating and evaluating the music therapy process it is not surprising that it has been a slow and sometimes frustrating progress, and one which has had to find its feet alongside the growth of the profession as a whole. What is clear now is that research and practice can be complementary to each other, and that the profession will find further strength and confidence from being able to defend itself on its own terms. But this must be on the basis of sustained enquiry which comes from asking appropriate questions about the work.

Some of the 'first generation' researchers in music therapy emerged somewhat disillusioned from their experiences and with warnings to colleagues. Having collaborated with researchers from other disciplines (typically psychologists or medical researchers) they often found that the research methodology was inappropriate to their music therapy work – in short that it omitted what the music therapist saw as central, in the process of needing to quantify results and present them within a traditional research design. For example, in an article entitled 'Measurement Problems in Applied Music Therapy Research' (Adams 1987) in the *Journal of British Music Therapy* the advice given is to ignore what happens within the musical process and concentrate on finding ways of measuring what happens outside it – in whatever aspect of physiological or psychological behaviour the music therapist wishes to change.

To many music therapists this solution is unsatisfactory to them: both as therapists and musicians. It leaves out from the research what they consider to be most important to their therapy, and tilts the therapeutic intent perilously close to behaviour modification. These kind of problems have led a second generation of music therapist researchers to investigate a broader scope of research strategies such as 'qualitative' and 'new paradigm' research and approaches which have evolved from studies in complementary medicine (Forinash 1993, Reason and Rowan 1981, Aldridge and Lewith 1993). For music therapy this involves respecting aspects of the scientific method without needing to be constrained by it, and searching for how to place centrally rather than peripherally the primary locus of music therapy – the *aesthetic* and personal within the musical. The challenge is still to find an appropriate research methodology consistent with how the therapy is seen to work, and which is sensitive enough to evaluate and validate this. These qualifications are not an attempt by music therapists to evade accountability but to ensure first that any evaluation is not based on criteria and methodology alien to its mode and field of operation. As David Aldridge writes, 'For a research methodology in the creative arts we cannot always revert to the questionnaire and the standard medical test. What we are challenged to develop is a way of presenting the work of art itself as it appears in the context of therapy' (Aldridge 1993b).

PROCESS VERSUS OUTCOME: QUALITY VERSUS QUANTITY

The underlying conflict in music therapy research lies between two sets of polarised concepts: quality–quantity and process–outcome. The first of these will I think now be clear. The second concerns the issue in the last section: the choice between investigating what happens *within* the musical process as against trying to measure aspects of the presumed result of this on the client (which need involve no musical aspect). Moreover quality–process and quantity–outcome tend to go together in pairs within music therapy research. One of the problems may be that these pairings and the thinking behind them have themselves become polarised and stuck. It is becoming clearer, on the contrary, how process and outcome work are related – and that we need preparatory work into the smallest details of the therapeutic work itself in order to be able to ask the right questions: so that any 'outcome' study can have meaning and validity to both therapists and clinicians.

Idries Shah tells a Sufi story in which, at a border pass, customs officials were puzzled for years by an old man they suspected of smuggling on his frequent trips over the border on his donkey. Repeated searches found nothing and eventually, in exasperation, they offered him clemency in exchange for an answer to the mystery.'So what are you smuggling?' they asked.'Donkeys,' he said.

In just this way the 'givens' of any technique are often too close to be seen and, consequently, 'process' research is needed to take a closer, analytic look at what practitioners do both consciously and unconsciously as a result of their technique, experience and professional instinct. The earlier chapter of this book 'Just a Minute...' is process research in a small way. The questions it asks are, what exactly is happening within the second-to-second process of this approach? and, is it possible to ascertain more closely *how* the process works, what is the catalyst of the therapeutic work, by looking more closely at *what* actually happened musically? This involves looking afresh at the evidence; challenging if necessary received dogmas of the technique; finding an accurate yet communicable language of description and suitable methods of analysis to 'map the territory' under observation; and finding a suitable assessment procedure to compare both sessions with the same client, and similar work with another client (Ansdell 1991).

In Creative Music Therapy the 'territory' (the area where what is taken to be essential happens) is seen to be the music and the 'musical between' of the client and therapist. Process investigations therefore need to focus on how to describe, represent, analyse and compare this in as much of its depth and complexity as is possible. As the chapter 'Reflecting' showed, different schools of music therapy take varying attitudes towards the musical material – interpreting it according to different theoretical starting-points. A largely musical descriptive level is, however, a possible common reference to which other therapists and non-therapists can discuss the work. The correlations between this level and other interpretations can be seen metaphorically rather than 'proved' (Aldridge *et al.* 1990, Aldridge 1993c).

RESEARCH IN CREATIVE MUSIC THERAPY: TWO EXAMPLES

An example of 'process' research in Creative Music Therapy is Colin Lee's investigation of improvised music within a therapy context (Lee 1992). This involved finding appropriate methods to scrutinise the most subtle levels of how the music functioned in the therapy, using an eclectic variety of musicological analytic approaches, supported by subjective verbal comments on the music from the client, a musician and a counsellor. His work gives a representation of the depth and complexity of musical and creative interaction between therapist and client and how this kind of work can lead to further questions about the nature of the music therapy process.

Research needs the sustained microcosmic analysis of this area where, as Kenneth Aigen (1991) remarked, our intuitions tell us that what is central takes place. At the same time, investigation cannot stay with this microcosm if its purpose is to go beyond intellectual curiosity and be of some use to the profession as a whole. Detailed studies at the purely musical level focus the problems of communicating knowledge gleaned, given the central problem of talking about music therapy: the often awkward blend of descriptions in musical terminology mixed with concepts borrowed from a generalised therapeutic discourse. One of the next priorities in research must be towards clarifying how to communicate to other professionals the significance of insights into how the minutiae of the music-therapeutic process link to the aims, objectives and outcomes of the therapy. In this way the 'process' and 'outcome' viewpoints are not polarised but essentially connected. Moreover, the bridge between them consists of the language, concepts and methods used and developed in research.

'Outcome' research typically requires some demonstration that the purported aims of the therapy can be to some extent objectively demonstrated to be valid. If the therapy aims to bring about change within certain parameters, is this achieved, in what way and how? Further, is it possible to demonstrate that any change that *is* registered is done so by means of the central technique under study and not by some other more peripheral phenomenon? Consequently, 'outcome' studies are typically supported by a more quantitative methodology. For whilst qualitative research determines what kind of things there are to be investigated, quantitative work determines how many of these there are – their pervasiveness (Heyink and Tymskra 1993).

A research project done by music therapist Mercedes Pavlicevic (Pavlicevic 1991, Pavlicevic and Trevarthen 1989) goes some way to bridging the gap between 'process' and 'outcome' research in music therapy. The subject of her research – the interaction between music, emotion and communication[3] – tackles directly some of the claims made for music therapy as a treatment. But it manages to research this area through a methodology recognisable and acceptable to clinicians: without, however, devaluing the essence of the music therapy process. Her project (in conjunction with the psychologist Colwyn Trevarthen) used a hypothesis derived from 'process' research to lay the ground parameters for a comparative study of the improvised playing of three groups: fifteen schizophrenic patients, fifteen depressed patients and fifteen normal controls. The criterion for comparison was formalised in a self-developed scale designed to access the musical interaction between the therapist and client in the music, which is taken to demonstrate the level and quality of emotional contact each of the groups were able to make and sustain. In this study the methodology of assessment was clear, and the level of investigation moved outside of the domain of the purely internal operation of the musical process. Though not strictly quantitative, its descriptions and interpretations are accessible to other therapists and clinicians, and show how the purely musical assessment can generate extra-musical significance about a patient group (in this case emotional health and interactive contact).

Pavlicevic's work represents a valuable and necessary half-way house for music therapy research, developing a model of inter-subjective validity. This avoids total subjectivity, where the reference-point is indefinable, whilst being able to accommodate the very necessary *qualitative* perceptions of the therapist which cannot be measured or mechanically applied. An intersubjective evaluation should be able to be shared by people outside of any specific theory but who do share the basic assumptions of a culture.

---

3 The philosophical basis of this study was outlined in Chapter 15.

SINGLE CASES

It is perhaps unfair to caricature other professionals as demanding from music therapists only outcome studies and hard proof. Nevertheless, whilst 'does it work?' is often an inappropriate question, the gentler 'does it make a difference?' is perhaps reasonable. For it is surely in its basic reliability to initiate change that Creative Music Therapy 'qualifies' as a therapy, rather than as 'just' an alleviating activity. This difference need not be defined in terms of what the approach does not intend (such as verbal insights or symptomatic relief) but it needs to demonstrate how it provides a systematic approach to the client and his problems.

Thirty years ago Nordoff and Robbins developed assessment and evaluation scales for use with mentally handicapped and autistic children (Nordoff and Robbins 1977). The assumption behind this was of a correlation between changes seen in the music therapy (defined by musical and musical-relational parameters) and developmental change (music therapy seen as acting to motivate retarded development – motor, perceptual and language). Basing an evaluation of therapeutic change on these criteria, however, is inappropriate for much of work presented in this book with adults living with chronic illness or mental health problems.

What Creative Music Therapy can give to all its clients – children or adults, impaired or non-impaired – is a fundamentally similar quality of experience provided by music and a musical relationship. The effects of this experience can range from diversion and alleviation through to providing the basis for significant personal transformation. As a therapist I certainly work to some extent from a developmental premise on the purely musical level: encouraging the gradual unfolding and development of creative freedom and possibility in the music and in the musical relationship. With some clients this can be seen as a progressive and cumulative development between the sessions and over perhaps the years of work. With others clients, as some of the case studies in this book show (especially work with terminally ill clients), the significant change is not between the sessions, but *within* them and within the music – but only perhaps, in T.S. Eliot's phrase, 'while the music lasts...' Be it because of the nature of their problem or because of the limits of music therapy itself, an evaluation only in terms of 'before and after' criteria is often unfair to the nature of the process.

Where significant change does occur this needs investigation with as individual a method as is possible. David Aldridge, a medical researcher who has thoroughly investigated the problems of researching music therapy, advocates 'single-case designs' (Aldridge 1992, 1993b). These are, he writes, 'an attempt to formalise clinical stories'. They can be of flexible design, but typically randomise treatments rather than patients, whose subjective evidence is seen as both valid and valuable. Blind assessments are also used to try to link formally changes in the patient with effective treatments:

> Most of the previous research published in the medical literature [on music therapy] indicates, albeit indirectly, changes in the quality of life in patients and subsequent changes in depression... Single-case studies incorporating elements of both medical assessment and musical assessment can be an effective compromise, allowing for both individual treatment initiatives and consideration of scientific medicine. Small group trials can then be designed from understandings gleaned in the single-case investigations, which will elicit those parameters that are subject to measurement and assessment. Longitudinal studies, involving compared groups or matched controls, may be feasible at a later stage for comparing chronic problems that are either resistant to change or subject to long-term change. (Aldridge 1993b)

An implication of an increased respect given to individual and subjective data is that 'anecdotal evidence' be given greater weight. The development of adult work in Creative Music Therapy has meant that a new level of material is available to investigate the process. In contrast to the handicapped children the approach began with, many of our adult clients can give sometimes sophisticated comments and reports of their experience of the therapeutic process. This was an important aspect of Colin Lee's study, and throughout this book there are valuable comments from clients which generate a wealth of questions both for research and about research.

THE VALUES OF EVALUATION

In music therapy's relatively short history research strategies have followed both fashion and necessity. It may be, as Leslie Bunt suggests, that we have already come round full circle:

> The early anecdotal descriptions demonstrating music's almost innate power to do good evolved into a period of increased rigour. There was a striving for objectivity and much borrowing from well-established research methods. The development of outcome studies has been, for the most part, very much under the control of the researcher, with the various designs set up in response to different contexts and based upon the researcher's value system. This period has led in turn to a stage in which rigour is applied in both objective analysis and subjective self-reporting. (Bunt 1994)

Yet however justifiably we put increasing importance on the need for evaluation and research in music therapy, we must not forget that our clients come not to be measured or diagnosed but to create something expressively and to communicate it to another person. The central activity of the session is an aesthetic one, and what remains of the session on the tape afterwards is to an extent an aesthetic object. It is therefore not an explanation or a proof of anything, just another 'picture' of a person – which relies, like all art, upon inter-subjective understanding first and foremost. Moreover, clients' comments stand primarily as reports of experience – individual, subjective and imaginative thoughts and feelings – but most of all as statements of *value*. The word 'evaluating' is often used as a synonym for 'assessing' or other quantitative methods. But within the word itself is the notion of value – a *qualitative* element which has no place outside the world of individual cases, subjective judgements and unmeasurable phenomena. This is true for music in general and for music therapy in particular.

CHAPTER 25

Mathew

> Our tests, our approaches, I thought, as I watched her on the bench – enjoying not just a simple but a sacred view of nature – our approach, our 'evaluations', are ridiculously inadequate. They only show us deficits, they do not show us powers; they only show us puzzles and schemata, when we need to see music, narrative, play; a being conducting itself spontaneously in its own natural way. (Oliver Sacks)

In the interval of a fundraising event I was standing in front of a display board with photographs showing people in music therapy. 'I know that man – he's the conductor', said a woman looking closely at one of the photographs. She went on to describe in detail the events in a video of Mathew which I show at most of the talks I give on music therapy. It was somewhat of a blow to my ego that she had no idea when or where she had seen the video, nor had she any recollection of me or of anything I had said. But Mathew, and more especially Mathew's music, had stayed with her.

Mathew's story was not unusual. He was born with Down's Syndrome and had lived with his mother until her death a few years before. He had then found himself in the totally different environment of a community hostel for adults with special needs. The psychiatrist who referred Mathew to music therapy wrote, not surprisingly, of how difficult he had found it to cope both with this violent change in his life and with his grief over his parent's death. He had become depressed, withdrawn and occasionally aggressive.

Mathew had started work for a short time with another music therapist who for practical reasons had been unable to continue. She left some notes saying that Mathew came to the sessions infrequently and only when he was in a good mood. He would look heavy and depressed, though was usually willing to play music, and there were good signs of the beginning of a musical relationship. She described his playing as cautious and precise, with little expression, and that he mostly waited for some direction from the therapist.

When we began working with Mathew[1] roughly the same pattern continued for the first three months or so. He was a friendly, tubby man with a very gentle manner and a child-like smile. But though he seemed to enjoy the sessions he would only come at the most twice a month, which was frustrating since we never seemed to be able to build on anything. His key-worker explained that it was simply impossible to persuade Mathew to come if he was not in the right mood. Had we, he asked, not seen him stubborn or even aggressive yet?

The answer to this was no, and for that matter we never did in the following two-and-a-half years we worked with him. It became apparent quite soon that, in this and other ways, Mathew was somehow different in the music therapy sessions. Usually stumbling in his attempts to communicate with words (his vocabulary consisted of only a few stereotyped phrases), when playing music he suddenly gained fluency and skill. As a personality he was usually shy and passive, but he found confidence and assertiveness when communicating in music. Writing about this work now it seems less of a gradual development than a case of contrasts: of describing the expected against the unexpected, the habitual against the transcendent (and I do not use this word lightly). Looking back I am often thinking, 'Usually he did this, but then this happened...' His potential would fly out from his limitations at unexpected moments. He was both limited and unlimited, conditioned and unconditioned, stuck and utterly free. This account attempts to describe the background against which two particularly important episodes happened.

'Nice weather, today?' Mathew would comment at the beginning of every session (even in deepest winter), and we would sing hello to each other. This became increasingly protracted given that Mathew demanded a diplomatic exactitude in who sang to who (there being six possible combinations with the three of us). He seemed to enjoy the ritual elements of the session but was equally happy, right from the beginning, improvising freely with his voice or on the instruments. Though a heavily built and powerful man he could play with delicacy and precision, his attention absorbed in what he

---

1 'We' being myself and Cheow Godfrey, who began working within a traditional role of 'co-therapist'. This, as we shall see, changed.

was doing. I noted in the first session how he could sustain a pulse, sense changes in tempo and construct his own rhythmic patterns. What was also noticeable was his almost immediate recognition of the communicative side of playing music together. He showed an openness and an enjoyment in the dialogue[2] which we established almost immediately in the music. On the other hand, Mathew was less happy taking initiative in the improvisations, waiting for the therapists to make any change. We also noticed that, after a while, he would often get stuck in his own playing – in a recurring rhythmic or melodic pattern. At this point we seemed to lose the sense of communication in the music, and he seemed to stop listening to the 'outside', getting drawn trance-like into his own repetitive action.

This also perhaps had something to do with my side of the music-making, since if what I played on the piano was too vague or too musically complicated I would lose Mathew. On the other hand when the music was right for him he became creative and emotionally involved. In the first session a Blues-like style got him clicking his fingers and whistling. When the music was right for him he responded with his whole body, often asking Cheow whether she would dance with him when just playing was not enough.

Things went smoothly for four sessions. Apart from the apparent ease with which he had accepted us and the situation there was nothing out of the ordinary. We worked in a fairly conventional way to encourage Mathew to listen as well as to play, to become more aware of how the music-making worked between the three of us, and how to limit his tendency to get stuck in perseverative rhythms. The staff at the hostel where Mathew lived said that he was excited by the music therapy sessions and tried to talk about them.

Then, quite unexpectedly, he refused to come four weeks in a row. His key-worker told us that he was having violent mood-swings, but when I went to visit Mathew was as friendly as usual. He seemed happy to come to music therapy again and we arranged that he would come the next Monday morning – which was exactly what he did, with no hint that there had been any break.

We carried on, and again there was nothing especially remarkable in the following months – though there was certainly a steady increase in our mutual enjoyment of the sessions and a deepening of the musical relationship. We encouraged Mathew to play melodic instruments (a metalophone, or a

2 It was more of a 'trialogue' really: Mathew enjoyed the three-way musical communication between us. He did not need Cheow as co-therapist to help him physically, but he did need her as an additional musical voice.

piano duet with me) and it was clear how good a sense of melody and phrasing he had. He also loved to sing, either improvising or in lengthy prolongations of our hello and goodbye songs. The latter often grew out of the style of the previous improvisations, and it was clear that there were certain musical idioms in which Mathew was at his most creative and responsive: mostly slow jazz or hymn-like styles. He was moved by these in all senses – he seemed to have a real instinct for 'soul' in music.

My intuition of this was amply confirmed just five months after we had started working together – in the first of what I have called the 'episodes'. Before one of Mathew's sessions I set up the video cameras (on a whim rather than a plan) having made a video of only one of his sessions previously. As a result I managed to catch a one-off event that could not have been captured on the usual audio-tape: it quite literally needs to be seen to be believed. It also stands as my most treasured evidence of what can happen in a free and creative music therapy, when the unexpected develops quite naturally out of the expected. The following attempt to describe in words what happened in that five minutes must, however, be accompanied by the proviso that what is both amazing and disquieting lies in the detail and the atmosphere rather than the 'facts' of the incident.

The three of us were sitting around the piano improvising vocally. As the music became animated Mathew started waving his hands, then stood up and took from the top of the piano a drumstick which he began to use as a baton. We continued singing, though the music I played on the piano became quicker and stronger – a regular pulse of chords against which we syncopated our voices. Mathew seemed acutely aware and involved, beating time with deft movements of his 'baton', his body swaying with the music. He had presumedly watched conductors on the television, but even so this was obviously no play-act – his beat was precise and controlled. Looking back at the video I realise that in the first few minutes I take control of the music, assuming perhaps that Mathew is 'just' beating time. Consequently I made the first change: slowing suddenly, though Mathew picked this up instantly. In the next minute I teased him musically, making an accelerando in my playing then a sudden stop, which caught him out. He, however, repeated the same trick, making his own pause. It worked, and from this point he took charge of the music. Whether it was that Mathew realised he *could* control what was happening, or that I had stepped back sufficiently, is hard to tell.

He returned the music to a pulse and made a waving motion of his baton in the air to 'compose' a tremolando in the music. I say 'compose' because it felt increasingly to me and Cheow from this point that Mathew knew what he wanted the music to be and was composing it on the spot through us, with precise instructions in the gestures of his hands and body. He then turned his back to me and conducted Cheow, moulding her singing into a slowing cadential figure. He brought her off precisely, with a slight bow, and again turned to me. After a second to collect the atmosphere he brought me in with the piano. This was when the real change in the piece happened. A totally different music emerged – I found myself singing a slow, hymn-like melody, accompanied by rich chords in E major, the style a cross between Bruckner and a Victorian hymn – giving an almost reverential atmosphere. It seemed perfect for Mathew, his body swaying as he conducted. But he was also firmly in control, letting me sing the first phrase, then bringing Cheow in for the second, the two dovetailing perfectly.

The music seemed to have found its style now, and sustained this until the end of the piece. Mathew continued to weave the music with the three elements he had at his disposal – Cheow's voice, my voice and the piano. With uncanny precision he would bring in a voice and shape the character and direction of the phrase with graceful but accurate gestures of his hands, then bring that voice off and another in, often overlapping the two by using both hands separately. And not only did his awareness focus on the two sometimes contrapuntal voices, but also seemed to include the harmonic character of the piano accompaniment.

Though at the time what happened seemed somehow right and inevitable, in retrospect it seems almost impossible to believe that a man so seemingly limited intellectually could call upon such awareness of the music and such precision of intention. It is important to see and hear that this was not just an act – a copying of a conductor's gestures. Rather Mathew seemed to have a precise intentional control over what happened in the music, and he was using his hands to compose the music he was unable to play for himself. The conductor Leonard Bernstein said that, in front of an orchestra he often felt he was re-composing the music. But Mathew had no score to start with – he was not re-composing, but composing. I believe that he knew what he wanted, musically and emotionally, and that we were merely giving sound to the form he was communicating to us.

Out of interest I wrote out what I could of the final section of the piece in musical notation, which revealed how clear and well balanced it was formally. I then watched the video again with the score and marked all the details of what I could see came directly as a result of Mathew's intention (through his conducted gestures), or those elements his awareness focused on and reacted to – trying as it were to follow his musical train of thought.

These points include details of phrasing, tempo, articulation, melodic direction and pauses. But also some of the harmonic details of voice-leading, which is far more surprising. There is no doubt at one point that Mathew senses the harmonic tension of a 9–8 suspension in the piano and conducts the resolution of this. What is remarkable is that, unlike the other details, this is not in the 'foreground' of the music (its obvious melody, phrasing, tempo, etc.) but part of its structural harmonic 'background', which would I think be seen to be inaccessible to someone academically untrained as a musician. It is these details which took place in a split second of time which are the core of the mystery of this episode.

Mathew shaped with care the final cadence, balancing and sustaining the two voices. On the last chord he raised both hands in the air, palms forward and kept them there until the music stopped, when he slowly lowered them and then his whole body in a slow bow. Cheow and I both clapped spontaneously.

Most groups I have shown this video to also spontaneously applaud at the end. It contains something very satisfying aesthetically as well as being a puzzle and a mystery on another level. A professional conductor who saw it remarked that Mathew's conducting was more technically competent than that of most of his colleagues!

This incident was a shock to us: it cut across the preconceptions we had built up about Mathew in the first six months. It was as if he was saying now 'You see me as this – but I'm *this* as well!' In music Mathew seemed to have found access to a depth, and we in turn had found access to the depth in Mathew. This was wonderful but not comfortable!

The week after the conducting episode I feared Mathew might try to repeat it yet fail to find the same experience. I should have known better – neither that week nor in the remaining two years we worked with him did he ever do anything similar. At the same time there was no overnight transformation in Mathew's 'everyday' playing. Instead there was a steady change in the next few years – the result of hard, steady work from all of us. There remained what I saw to be an ongoing battle between his creativity and getting stuck (which manifested mainly as 'perseveration'); between his limitations and his potential. After the conducting episode, however, we felt justified in making the sessions more of a challenge. An aspect of this was to set up the room differently – with the piano surrounded by an array of instruments – and encourage Mathew to be more active in his choice of instrument and rely on him to initiate and change the music.

At first tentative, he became increasingly adventurous and enjoyed the three-way improvisations, which he could sustain for fifty minutes almost non-stop. Our concentration and energy was often exhausted before his. At the purely musical level we tried to let Mathew help himself when he became stuck in heavy, repetitive rhythms or endless wandering melody. This involved resisting the desire to intervene musically ourselves in order to nudge him into changing, and instead to go along with the perseveration until some 'critical limit' at which point Mathew himself would mostly make a change of his own free will. Through this he experienced less musical dependency on us and more of his own ability to take initiative even when he had become stuck. He continued to get stuck of course, but also I think realised at some level that he could free himself and sometimes even transcend himself as he did in the two episodes.

At about this time the Speedwell Trust (who supported the music therapy unit we worked in) were making a fundraising video and asked whether it would be possible to film one of our sessions. I agreed with some trepidation since the intrusion of a camera (not to mention a whole film crew) can often be very intimidating for a client, awkward for the therapist, with the result looking artificial and strained. Mathew, however, had no such problems and was a true professional. He insisted on shaking hands with the whole film crew and then played unselfconsciously with all the spontaneity and involvement that he showed when only the three of us were there.

Watching the results of the filming later we were struck by just how different Mathew was from the man who had come only a year before. He now had an air of confidence and was obviously proud of himself and his music. When we met with Mathew's key-worker we heard similar reports concerning his life in general. He was seldom depressed now, he had more self-confidence and self-esteem and was less compliant and passive in his life. Though these changes were helped by the efforts of many people who were working with Mathew, it was clear that music therapy was very important to him and had a major influence at this time.

For another fairly long period our work together went steadily, with the occasional highs and lows you might expect from a process spanning years. There was another period when Mathew refused to come for a month. When I visited him I found that his home life had been disturbed again by staff changes (the third time in a year), and Mathew seemed upset and insecure. He came back to music, however, and continued as before, again as if nothing had happened.

Something did happen in the session on 22 April 1991, however. My usually sketchy notes for the sessions extend to five pages for that day. This was the second of the 'episodes':

Quite simply 'It' happened. I know Cheow and I felt roughly the same experience – I think I know that Mathew did as well. Suddenly 'It' was playing: the music, us, the room lifted – as if being taken up a vertical shaft. I felt the emotion overwhelming.

The client before Mathew cancelled, and then chatting together we forgot the time and were ten minutes late in collecting Mathew from the waiting room. I hadn't even prepared the instruments. Eventually we got down to the session and Mathew started playing a drum and cymbal near the piano. He seemed especially concentrated and committed in his playing today, even for Mathew. He took the lead to a large extent, changing the patterns and tempo of his playing quite frequently. I felt I was being kept on my toes, but also that Mathew was giving me quite precise 'instructions' as to the character of the music he wanted from me. This much of the session is on tape. The character of the music sounds quite forceful, heavy, hard even.

Cheow stood behind us listening. She said later that in the last few weeks she'd only played when and what Mathew asked her to, since he'd increasingly shown the ability to know what he wanted. I felt, nevertheless, her passive concentration on the music and that she had picked up the intensity in the atmosphere today. The dialogue between Mathew and I lasted about fifteen minutes. There was an incredibly close connection between us in the music – a real sharing of intention. But at the same time there was something of the feeling that we were both testing one another – that we were both trying too hard.

Mathew then indicated to Cheow that she should play the xylophone (which had a black-note pentatonic scale), so I changed key to accommodate the new voice. The tape has about thirty seconds of this change before running out. This almost seems symbolic, since the next ten minutes could not really exist on a tape. I can't describe it fully either, of course – it was a mystical experience in the sense that the whole was distinctly more than the sum of the parts, and the experience of the whole is all that really remains with me. Many things seemed to change at the same time: Mathew's drumming seemed to take on a different quality, changing from a heavy 'down' it became a source of 'up' energy, giving a sense of dance to the music. Around this Cheow and I 'danced' syncopated pentatonic melodies and cross rhythms. My feeling was of a sudden lightness of touch, a freedom from controlling the situation or determining the music. I remember looking down at my hands in disbelief and seeing them playing.

Everything seemed to lift – lightness is the only metaphor that seems accurate to describe the loss of effort and the joy of the playing. The other feeling was that though none of us was doing anything especially remarkable, that somehow the music had happened itself and had taken off and taken us with it! Suddenly all the parts seemed to connect and the music seemed to come through...

These are the only, not very satisfactory, terms I can explain this, the only experience of this type I've had in music therapy. It was genuinely beyond planning, controlling, and perhaps importantly, beyond individuals. The last time Mathew surprised us (with the conducting episode) we could still talk about our wonder at what *he*, Mathew, did. But this time I can't divide up the experience – it was more than any one of us, but at the same time included each of us totally. This was even more thrilling.

After two-and-a-half years of weekly sessions with Mathew we decided to think about coming to a close. The decision was a hard one, since we all enjoyed the sessions and there was no pressing reason to stop them, apart from having to find space for new clients. But at the same time we had the feeling that we had completed a circle with Mathew: that what had needed to happen *had* happened. Knowing, however, that in the past changes and losses had caused such disturbance for Mathew we prepared the end slowly and carefully. Mathew surprised me by suddenly saying 'three more left' at the end of a session. He was right, but I had never heard him say something that precise before. Our final session was not especially eventful. At the end we said goodbye and Mathew left, showing no more emotion than usual, though he was aware it was the last session. My ego perhaps would have appreciated a more obvious expression of loss. Cheow and I would, after all, miss Mathew and our music-making together. But this brought home to me one of the central points about music therapy with Mathew – that though I think he liked us as people, he was primarily there for the music and it was within the music that the significance of our work rested. Mathew found in the world of music and musical communication a way to create, to fulfil and occasionally to transcend himself and his limitations: to say 'Yes, I'm this – but I'm *also* "this"!'

POSTSCRIPT

In writing up case studies (especially ones like this) two doubts seep in. First that somehow you have made more of it than was really there, and second, that you exaggerate the significance of the hour a week in the music therapy room in relation to the 'real' life any of our clients live the remaining hours in the week. The first worry I can rationalise by accepting the basic subjectivity of the case study, but a subjectivity tempered by what we can see on a video, hear on a tape, or discuss with someone who also experienced something similar (my colleague Cheow in this instance, to whom I showed the first draft of this chapter). The second reservation concerns me more, and it is always heartening to know what happened to someone after you have stopped working with them.

After having written a first draft of this case study I met by chance Mathew's first key-worker, John, who had brought him along to the sessions for the first year or so. He had moved to a new job after this and had recently met Mathew by chance, some four years after he had first known him. He was happy to report that Mathew really was a changed man – happy and confident, going out with other residents to the pub, really enjoying life, in John's words. Music therapy was of course only one part of many different attempts to help Mathew. But nevertheless, from the nature of the experiences which Mathew had in music therapy, I cannot believe that it was not a significant part.

After much consideration I decided in the end not to include audiotape excerpts of Mathew's sessions. When selecting suitable material it was clear that this would not be fair to him. At the present state of technology at least, it was not possible to reproduce the conducting episode in a form which could go with this book. Additionally the second 'episode' I write about in this case was not (and perhaps could not be) on tape. Instead I have miles of tape of Mathew at what could be called his 'base-line' state: playing musically and often charmingly, but nothing like the 'apex' of his playing represented by the 'episodes'. To present the 'base-line' material without the 'apex' seemed unfair to Mathew. I hope nevertheless that the descriptions give enough of an idea of what happened – at least until the appropriate technology is available.

CHAPTER 26

Connecting

> By aesthetic I mean responsive to the pattern which connects. (Gregory Bateson)

It is tempting to leave Mathew's case as it stands, without comment – as a prime example of the individual instance I wrote about in 'Evaluating'. Furthermore, most of the aims and methods behind our work with Mathew were largely overshadowed by what was unexpected, unprepared for and, it would seem, unexplainable. Given this, it is perhaps not a case study to choose to draw any general principles from. Yet at the same time it was the work that posed the most questions to me about music, music therapy and the relationship between the two – a preoccupation which has remained central to this book. If we are not just to exclude Mathew from discussion on the grounds of him being somehow a unique case, then the questions his case poses may perhaps lead into some interesting areas, if not to any conclusive answers. My hunch was that the more unusual aspects of this work were pointing towards some important characteristics of the process of Creative Music Therapy in general, rather than to something which had just a one-off significance. Moreover, some of the issues it raises seem to form a focus for the connections between the other cases, and between these and the essays on aspects of the process. This final chapter, then, offers some connections by way of a conclusion.

'KNOW HOW' AND 'KNOW THAT'

Our society often defines people's mental ability (and often worth) with a quantitative measure, their IQ. Mathew's score was representative of the trouble he had with language and handling abstract thought. Yet this same man, in the conducting episode in particular (but also at many other times), showed a level of sophistication and subtlety in music which totally belied the usual implication of his so-called 'intelligence quotient'.

Oliver Sacks makes the same point in reference to people he got to know and wrote about. One boy he calls the 'Autist Artist':

> His mind is not built for the abstract, the conceptual. *That* is not available to him as a path to truth. But he has a passion and a real power for the particular – he loves it, he enters into it, he re-creates it. And the particular, if one is particular enough, is also a road – one might say nature's road – to reality and truth. (Sacks 1985)

But how concrete, how 'particular' really is music? Many people, thinking perhaps of the complexity of much music, would say that it is quite an abstract thing – difficult, after all, even to describe. And certainly much of the argument of this book has been that music *can* stand on its own – not referring directly to things in the world, even necessarily to our own emotional states. Moreover, Mathew's grasp of music in the episodes was anything but simple – he very definitely was not just riding on a current of feeling. He showed instead an uncanny and certainly intentional control over some very subtle details of musical construction and expression, which he was able to convey to us through gesture. But it is perhaps precisely in this last fact that a possible answer lies. Mathew's music was not the abstraction of a score, but *the thing itself* – the musical phenomenon unfolding on the crest of its own logic, yet intimately related to his own bodily and emotional perceptions. Yet at the same time this did not exclude complexity of intention and execution.

What we sometimes forget in Western music is that it is the score which is abstract, not the music when it is played. We forget, in Korzybski's phrase, that 'The map is not the territory – the name is not the thing named' (1941). In reference to this idea, Gregory Bateson (1980) comments that the two sides of the brain handle the respective functions of the concrete and the abstract, and that 'the symbolic and affective hemisphere is probably unable to distinguish name from thing named'. This was doubtless true of Mathew, who had a practical and imaginative, but not a conceptual grasp of music. He could feel the direction of the melody, the shape of the phrasing, the movement of the rhythms, the tensions of the harmony – not I think sensed from 'outside' the music but somehow felt 'within' or 'alongside' it. Yet he was unable to abstract this into words or notes or concepts, the reality of the music being to him in the concrete here-and-now of the improvisation. The same was also true of David and what I described earlier as his empirical discovery of the elements and the constructive and expressive principles of music. Though David had more verbal ability than Mathew, he equally had no *conceptual* grasp of his playing – he discovered, but did not 'know' the rules of harmony and counterpoint. He had, in Gilbert Ryle's phrase 'know-how' rather than 'know-that' (Ryle 1971) – arguably an advantage over many cerebral Western musicians. For after all 'music, at root, is what musicians know how to do' (Elliott 1993).

MUSICALITY

Perhaps what best describes what Mathew showed at these moments is 'musicality' – a quality which involves both 'musical thinking' (or 'know-how'), and 'musical feeling'. It is sometimes implied that the Mathews and Davids of this world are limited to the latter, only reacting to music rather than being able to 'understand' it. On the contrary I believe that Mathew and David's musicality involved significant 'musical thinking' – by which I mean: an ability to control musical intentions; to give form and meaning to sound; to create something coherent in the world of music.

A further question is whether this 'musical thought' can be credited as 'real' thought – or, put another way, is there such a thing as non-logical, non-conceptual/propositional thought? Socrates, Goethe and Heidegger, to call three not inconsiderable witnesses, believed so – and Zuckerkandl considers this is a vital point in understanding the nature of the musical experience:

> There is, then, such a thing as logical thinking, thinking in concepts, and there is such a thing as musical thinking, thinking in motions. Conceptual thinking leads to judgements, musical thinking to tonal patterns. Every concept is a concept 'of' something, a reflection of reality. Motion is real in itself. Conceptual thinking is cognitive, its purpose to add to our store of knowledge. Musical thinking is productive, its purpose to add to our store of reality. Conceptual thinking owes its internal order to the laws of logic which govern it: it is natural to assume that musical, productive thinking owes its internal order to laws of its own. (Zuckerkandl 1973)

'Musical thinking' is no less real than the verbal-conceptual thinking which IQ tests measure, and with which people like Mathew have such trouble. But, as Oliver Sacks comments, this is mostly the *only* type of thinking evaluated. In order to do justice to people as a whole, and to explain some of the nature of these different skills, clearly a wider concept of 'thought' itself is required.

Novalis wrote 'In the painter the hands become a locus of an instinct, and the same is true of the musician.' Thinking in music is not a problem-solving, but a productive and creative mode of thought which takes its meaning from gestures and bodily feelings as well as from the feedback from the medium itself (the connection between the tones and the musician's ears and hands) – the procedure described in the earlier chapter 'Creating'. Whilst the conceptual thinker stands back from what he works with, the 'productive' thinker stands somehow *in* whatever she is creating. In this way somehow doing is inseparable from thinking. Again Zuckerkandl explains this well, writing about the process of improvisation:

> The inner ear and inner hand must be one breath ahead of the outer ear and outer hand...the notes seem to meet the hand half-way, as though of their own volition, yet we feel the presence of something else which guides the hand from within! The sounds have become an expressive gesture...the tones themselves have become hand, since they speak in gestures. (Zuckerkandl 1973)

This describes beautifully what seems to be happening when I look at the video of Mathew's conducting episode: where there is no firm line between what leads and what follows – the music or the gestures; between new inspiration or the following of the implications unfolding from the pattern already there.[1]

These issues are relevant, moreover, not just to music therapy with clients with learning difficulties. They bring into relief a double aspect of all of our experiences of music. People like Mathew, Emanuella, Tom and Jack have no choice but to experience music concretely and 'purely musically'. Other music therapy clients (especially trained musicians) also have another mode of approaching music: they are, we could say, adept with the map as well as the territory of music, having learned to conceptualise and abstract it, to read scores, to analyse and talk about it. For them Creative Music Therapy, with its emphasis on improvisation and direct communication, can perhaps give an opportunity to find the same mode of musical experience as Mathew and David: where 'musical thinking' is grounded in 'doing', and on an intimate personal connection with the music (Merleu-Ponty's 'complicity' with it).

If, then, there really is a purely musical mode of thinking which is accessible in ways different to what we usually call 'thought', what is it like?

---

1 See David Sudnow's (1978) account of learning to play jazz piano, *Ways of the Hand: The Organisation of Improvised Conduct.*

'THE PATTERN WHICH CONNECTS'

A starting suggestion in the argument of this book was that we ourselves are, like music, essentially 'patterned frequencies in time' (Aldridge 1989a). In the quotation above Zuckerkandl made the distinction between 'conceptual thought' leading to judgements (and I may add concepts, propositions, proofs, discoveries, implications), and 'musical thought' leading to 'tonal patterns'. Both musical perception and production have been shown by psychologists of music to be formidable skills of pattern perception and pattern-making, requiring complex cerebral mechanisms. Despite this there is still some reluctance to consider musical thought as being a similar status to 'real' (that is, verbal/conceptual/propositional) thought. But think back (perhaps play again the example) to the chapter 'Just a Minute...' and its demonstration of the musical and music-therapeutic process in microcosm. From nothing (and the client's expectation of nothing) grew something, as the music seemed to find its own connections and meaning in a constant metamorphosis of the given material. It referred *inside* itself rather than making connections with the world 'outside'. It had, like most music, the feel of something growing rather than constructed, of a patterning and elaboration which, though directed to an extent by a rule-governed, syntactical system, is nevertheless essentially unique and free in its creation and development. Additionally, in this example not only did the music seem to find connections within itself, it also made a connection *between* the client and therapist through the shared musical meaning they found in the 'musical between'. This is, of course, a vital aspect of the music-therapeutic process, but one which rests on a basic characteristic of how music works in general.

In the epigraph to the chapter on Mathew I quoted Oliver Sacks' comment about the fact that we often measure the deficits of a person but ignore their powers. Sacks was writing about his patient Rebecca, who herself used the metaphor of a pattern in describing herself and her needs:

> She looked down at the office carpet and said: 'I'm a sort of living carpet. I need a pattern, a design like you have on that carpet. I come apart, I unravel unless there's a design.' I looked down at the carpet, as Rebecca said this, and found myself thinking of Sherrington's famous image, comparing the brain/mind to an 'enchanted loom', weaving patterns, ever-dissolving, but always with meaning. I thought: can one have a raw pattern without a design... A 'living carpet' as Rebecca was, had to have both – and she especially, with her lack of schematic structure (the warp and woof, the *knit* of the

carpet, so to speak), might indeed unravel without a design (the scenic or narrative structure of the carpet). (Sacks 1985)

It was the quality of music as a 'living pattern' on both small and large scale which was the subject of the earlier chapter 'Recalling', where we saw how music made contact with Herr G. through the disorientation of a comatose state; gave Jack a sense of mental and physical connection when playing; gave Clive Wearing some anchor in time to knit together his unravelling consciousness. These examples show that the musical 'pattern' should not be thought of as something cold and abstract, but in fact the opposite: concrete, accessible and personal.

The one thing that a pattern is not necessarily is *representational* – and this may direct us to where the problem lies for many people in thinking of music as a 'patterned frequency in time' or saying that one of the central activities of Creative Music Therapy is pattern-making. It can sound inhuman or, at worst, simply trivial. Are we really comparing music to a kaleidoscope, or music therapy to joint carpet-weaving?

Peter Kivy, in an essay called *The Fine Art of Repetition* (Kivy 1993) reminds us of the enduring tension since the seventeenth century between two rival views of music. The first sees music as having a content and representing human emotions, speech, ideas (even if non-verbally). On the contrary the other view sees music essentially as contentless patterning (the so-called 'wallpaper analogy'), primarily as a decorative rather than a fine art. Perhaps not surprisingly, vestiges of the same argument can be found in the case of music therapy, with the different theories taking music to be more or less representational or more or less abstract. As polar opposites neither theory is likely to represent the whole truth for a situation as complex as a music therapy session, involving as it does both musical and personal considerations. Kivy's argument, however, is that what he calls the 'fallen theory', the 'musical wallpaper' analogy, deserves more serious consideration, and is not necessarily a trivialisation of the art of music (or, I might add, of the art of music as therapy). Music is a complex, dynamic pattern in sound, with its own grammar and its own mode of expression,[2] and as such represents in Kivy's view 'the redeeming of the decorative arts from the Western prejudice for knowing as the only goal worthy of the human intellect' (Kivy 1993).

---

2 This expression, however, can be a phenomenological *property* of the music: it is not necessarily a representation of the composer or performer's personal emotional state, nor does it necessarily arouse the same emotion in the hearer.

In the earlier chapter 'Reflecting' I put forward an argument against the assumption that the music in a music therapy session is exclusively a representation of the thoughts, feelings and images from the client's inner world – which consequently need verbal interpretation as part of the therapeutic process. Instead I suggested that the therapist in Creative Music Therapy makes what I called an 'intrinsic interpretation' of the music, responding creatively *within* the pattern of the music itself, helping the client to articulate herself musically and to communicate within music. This does not necessarily lead to new knowledge in the usual (verbal-conceptual) sense, but rather something new is found within the experience of being part of the creative growth and development of the music, an experience shared between therapist and client. This 'pattern which connects' can be one of real depth, meaning and beauty. It may be that, as Anthony Storr suggests, we undervalue the influence of the so-called abstract on our psychological well-being, 'The human mind seems so constructed that the discovery or perception of order or unity in the external world is mirrored, transferred and experienced as if it were a discovery of a new order and balance in the inner world of the psyche' (Storr 1988).

BUT IS IT ART? THE AESTHETICS OF MUSIC THERAPY

Is 'therapeutic art' Art with a capital 'A'? If so, then do normal aesthetic standards apply? If not, is beauty no part of it? Surprisingly, beauty also seems to be a 'fallen theory' in the arts therapies. Surprisingly, that is, since every one of the arts therapies grew out of its respective fine art, where aesthetic considerations are generally the only considerations. Yet Picasso himself made the inauspicious remark that 'the work of a madman is a dead work' (Thomson 1989). Jung and many subsequent psychodynamically oriented arts therapists, (also anthroposophic 'artistic therapies') seem not to have regarded the client's work as 'real' art, but as something for another purpose – be this an exercise or a screen for interpretation. In her book on art therapy Martina Thomson (1989) quotes the saying of her mentor, E.M. Lydiatt, on her patients work: 'Leave it flat – it is not art!' Perhaps this attitude can be explained by the emphasis the arts therapies have put on the *process* above the product in their justification of the clinical rigour of their discipline. Perhaps it was also a fear of being sentimental. Beauty, for whatever reason, is seldom mentioned as an element of the therapy.

Yet I do not think that the moments of beauty which happened in the music within the case studies in this book rested on sentimentality. They were, on the contrary, important – perhaps transformative – moments of the therapy, and they happened in 'real music' which *was* in my view Art with a capital 'A'. Colin Lee's client, Francis, said about improvising music together:

> There's no conscious process, I love it, this is what I dream of. And when something musically happens and you smile, and I think it's beautiful, it works, it's there, and it was something that just happened...I needed to express something and that's what came out, and it was right and it was beautiful.

The same could be said of Mathew's conducting episode, or David's solo on the electronic keyboard, or of moments in the group. In each case we were not consciously trying to make 'beautiful music' – it simply, and mostly unexpectedly, happened. These moments are preserved on the tapes of the sessions, and some reproduced on the CD with this book. As well as being a record of a clinical music therapy session, this music is also an aesthetic object in its own right – and any full understanding of it, as music therapy, demands also an aesthetic understanding. For, from this experience of the client(s) and therapist creating something beautiful, there was often some 'reflection' of a therapeutic significance. Recognising that they could create something beautiful (whether as an individual or a group) gave a sense of satisfaction, pride and self-worth. It is therefore impossible to address these issues of the aesthetic in Creative Music Therapy without them becoming a legitimate aspect of the therapeutic endeavour itself. The American philosopher Robert Grudin wrote, 'Beauty oddly resembles gravity: like gravity, beauty is a force whose existence is inferred from its apparent effects. You might even call beauty a kind of "spiritual gravity", a natural force of attraction, cohesion' (Grudin 1990).

This idea is closer to how I have looked at the other aspects of Creative Music Therapy such as 'meeting', 'quickening', 'creating': not as things in themselves but as processes which can largely be seen from their effects, and as such are phenomena which are part of musical *experience*. Given, then, an aesthetic element can be recognised in music therapy it is likely that it holds some significance within the therapeutic process. Beauty can be both a property *and* a process. Were it not such an ugly word we could perhaps add 'beautying' to the list of processes in Creative Music Therapy.

A colleague was once told, as something of a put-down, by a music therapist of another persuasion that *her* approach (unlike that of Creative Music Therapy) was not just about 'playing prettier and prettier tunes'. On the contrary, what I am talking about in this section is far from 'prettiness' and far from any intention of the music therapist to work for musical beauty as an end in itself. Grudin's 'spiritual gravity' or Rilke's 'terrible beauty' is nearer to the phenomenon I am trying to describe. It will, I hope, be clear from the case studies that this is exactly *not* a surface prettiness but a beauty achieved at some depth, often through the reconciliation of conflicting elements.

The traditional yardstick of the beautiful in music involves a balance between form and feeling: the formal qualities of unity, integration and coherence balanced against expressive authenticity and taste. These parameters seem also to be fundamental to the beautiful in music therapy as well. Francis talks of how 'it was something that just happened...I needed to express something and that's what came out, and it was right and it was beautiful'. He and others talk of the 'rightness' or the 'fit' of a moment of beauty which, far from being fabricated, just happened. This difference is partly a quality of improvisation, which means that in a music therapy session beauty is a quality which can happen *between* people, not just a quality of a musical object. It follows that the potential for the aesthetic is reliant to an extent on the quality of the musical relationship between therapist and client. If the nature of the musical relationship is one of freedom, trust and quality, so can the music which is the manifestation of this relationship. Beauty 'happens' because the whole situation is right. Equally the influence of these moments of beauty will strengthen and deepen the musical relationship.

The quality of the music as a whole is also very dependent on the quality of the therapist's music.[3] This is a contentious issue in music therapy as a whole for, if aesthetics are not seen to be an essential part of the therapeutic process, then the quality of music, or the quality of the musical competence of the therapist, is not such an issue.[4] In Creative Music Therapy, however, it is taken to be axiomatic that, whoever the client is – a handicapped child or a professional musician – they deserve the highest quality and sensitivity of music and music-making, one that can be defined and verified on aesthetic standards held by the musical profession as a whole.

The epigraph I chose for this chapter was Gregory Bateson's famous definition 'By aesthetic I mean responsive to the pattern which connects' (Bateson 1980). In his work across a wide variety of disciplines he tried to show how the aesthetic gives us an intuition of the unity and fundamental

---

3 Normally there is a discrepancy of musical skill between therapist and client, where the therapist is the trained musician playing the piano, and with most of the responsibility for the aesthetic quality of the music. This is, of course, not true when the client is a musician as well.

4 By 'quality' and 'competence' I do not mean complexity or aestheticism for its own sake. It is as much a matter of sensitive listening as playing.

connections between things: whether a Mozart symphony, the structure of a leaf or the complexities of human communication. He repeatedly came back to the concept of the aesthetic (in which he included pattern, metaphor and symbol, creativity, dream, myth) as the link between the natural and the human world, between thinking and feeling, creating and knowing. It is absolutely *not* a doctrine of 'prettiness', but an understanding of shared meaning and value in the world. Music itself is a prime example of 'the pattern which connects' – a phenomenon whose coherence and order within itself in turn connects people together through their shared responsiveness to it (whether in their perception of, or creation within, the pattern). In this sense the aesthetic has to be, in Creative Music Therapy, an essential part of the whole process.

MUSIC THERAPY AS PERFORMANCE

At the end of Mathew's conducting episode Cheow and I applauded spontaneously. If I ask myself why, I come to the idea that it was because it was, in a sense, a fine performance. Yet the idea of performance would seem to sit uncomfortably with most of the main features and tenets of therapy: as a private and largely introspective business concerned with authenticity and precisely *not* the 'acting a part' which the concept of performance can suggest. In several talks I have given on music therapy, however, I have used the idea of performance to investigate some of the implications of Mathew's case and other characteristics of Creative Music Therapy. I borrowed some ideas from a small book called *Performance* by the lutenist Anthony Rooley (1990). His appeal is not to the modern notion of performance, which is a development from the Romantic notion of the self-expressive artist projecting his ego through the music. Instead Rooley suggests a re-examination of the forgotten sixteenth-century understanding of performance based on neo-Platonic ideas. This gives a theory of the different levels of musical experience, before and within performance, and rather than involving an enhancement of the ego works for the opposite – where getting yourself *out* of the way allows the music and the dynamics of the performance to channel what is potential, unexpected and, ultimately, spiritual.

The first stage is called 'Decoro', the level of learned skill, the drudge element. But within a performance situation (whether just playing to someone else or to a thousand) something else comes into play – 'Sprezzatura' – which involves playing (in all senses) with the possibilities of the moment, what Rooley calls 'calculated carelessness'. Any improvisatory element is a prime example of this state, where there can be an extra energy which motivates and helps something new happen. But both of these levels are not ideally ends in themselves but prepare the ground for 'Grazia', an aesthetic and spiritual dimension which the sixteenth-century theorist Ficino described as something between 'divine frenzy' and 'sublime tranquility'. Rooley adds that, '"Grazia" is uncontrollable, unknowable, belonging to no one; but its presence is instantly recognisable... "Grazia" is channelled...it cannot be claimed, but there is no doubt that certain performances may be a channel for this rarest of human experience' (Rooley 1990). When I write in Mathew's case study in the second 'episode' that 'It' happened, this was, I think, an experience of 'Grazia'. Similarly, in the conducting episode Mathew seemed to be somehow borrowing our 'Decoro' (our learned technical ability as trained musicians) and the 'live' situation of the session gave a measure of 'sprezzatura'. But just occasionally we found access to the third level, which the theory sees as the legitimate goal of all performance, and where people can transcend the habitual and find a level of energy, motivation and concentration which can allow the unexpected to happen. When they are, in a word, *inspired.*

Performance is a natural context for music-making and a natural part of musical experience. 'Inspiration' is perhaps the modern equivalent of the concept of 'grazia', and I have found that a surprising number of people use the word 'inspiring' either to describe an experience of music therapy or of that of watching or hearing tapes of the process. That there is often an element of performance in the process of Creative Music Therapy is not to contradict its therapeutic aspect. A good performance is, after all, not an inauthentic 'show', but something where the conditions have given rise to an enhancement of the performer's ability and inspiration. So too with Creative Music Therapy, where the context gives an energy and an encouragement of potential.

Performance means literally 'through the form', and this thought leads back to the statement made by music therapist Mercedes Pavlicevic (1992), regarding her research into 'dynamic forms' in music: that the music therapy process gives people a chance for 'trying out new forms'. In the chapter 'Expressing' I quoted Suzanne Langer's argument against the belief that in playing music we are simply expressing ourselves. She reminded us that, in many cases, music can present emotions we have *not* felt before. So too in music therapy where the purely musical experience can give access to new forms of feeling, and new feelings of form – be this the new physical vista Karl discovered or the new emotional and social ones found by Emanuella, Charlie, Herr P., Gisela and Mathew. As another client once said to me 'For just an hour a week you showed me another "me".' This woman had a psychological illness where she believed herself to have multiple sclerosis.

She exhibited the physical symptoms of the illness and her social and emotional life had diminished in parallel to her physical problems. In her music therapy sessions, however, the music often unexpectedly 'moved' her and she found the seed of a new way of experiencing herself – that she could dare to 'try on a new form'. For her it involved letting go of some of the excessive self-control she imposed on herself. For another person, however, music therapy could give exactly the opposite – an experience of being able to make order, coherence and beauty in something; to find control.

Creative Music Therapy is not a symptomatic treatment, but an individual artistic pursuit. What the music therapist *can* do is to meet each person individually in music, and find a way of making music with them. The flexibility music has to make contact in the first place is also the flexibility it has to give the person playing the experience of 'trying on a new form'. Music never forces or coerces: it offers itself as a possibility. Creative Music Therapy mobilises this within a specialised context.

THE FACES OF MUSIC

Music has many faces and many uses. It has perhaps never been the single art we sometimes imagine, and happily holds many opposites in tension. Both Pythagorean science and expressive art; the Greek's amalgam of music and words ('musike') and the most non-verbal of the modern arts; a vehicle for direct emotional catharsis and the ultimate abstract form; a supremely social art and the most solitary introspective pleasure.

Given that music therapy is one of music's newest incarnations, it is not surprising that it has inherited most of these paradoxes. The various approaches to music therapy seem to take their emphases from these different faces of music, as well as from whatever pre-existing model of therapy they are allied to.

Creative Music Therapy is no exception to this, with its own emphasis being on the formal and phenomenological aspects of the musical experience rather than any explicit discussion of the emotional or symbolic dimensions. This, however, is not to say that these are excluded from the work. Indeed common sense tells us that music cannot exist without an emotional dimension. Form does not exclude feeling – indeed perhaps, as the French philosopher Dufrenne wrote, 'Feeling is the soul of form.' The point is that *talking* about feeling in music is not the same as experiencing an emotional dimension within the music. Talking about music is as much about words as it is about music, and it is this verbal-conceptual dimension which is largely avoided in the approach of Creative Music Therapy. The old analogy of music as a patterning of form has become unfashionable in our more expressionist culture, where every artistic act must become an expression of ourselves, to be de-coded subsequently by interpretation. There is still room, however, for the compensatory picture of the arts and the arts therapies as form-making activities in which we can build and find as well as just expressing. Music in particular, as the most abstract of the arts can fruitfully be relieved of some of the burden of always having to *represent* something, to carry extra-musical meanings. Yet music, paradoxical art that it is, can be both 'nothing but tones' whilst also the art which moves us most. Music therapy's power rests precisely on this fact.

THE FACTS OF THE MUSICAL EXPERIENCE

The music-making that music therapy gives access to rests on what Zuckerkandl (1959) called 'the facts of the musical experience'. These 'facts' do not emerge from any theory but from the practice of music-making, whether this be in a professional or an amateur setting, or in a music therapy room. I have tried to build up through the case studies and the essays of this book a collection of observations about these 'facts'. A summary might include the following:

- the concreteness and accessibility of music
- that doing and thinking cannot be separated in music
- that feeling and thinking cannot be separated
- that creativity, expressivity and beauty are its natural processes
- that music possesses unique qualities to quicken, give orientation and order the mind and the body
- that performance is a natural context of music-making
- that communication is its natural result.

Inclusive of all these there are perhaps two over-arching facts which support the principle of Creative Music Therapy. First that music is grounded in the body, in its processes and its expressions. Music is sympathetic to the whole self: we do not merely play or listen to music but *become music* while the music lasts, living both in it and through it. In T.S. Eliot's famous line, 'you are the music/while the music lasts'. It is this intimate connection between music and the patterns of our bodies, emotions and thoughts which is a fact of musical experience music therapy works with to give new experiences of feeling and form.

The second 'fact' is perhaps more essential than this even: that music lives *between* people; it makes contact, communicates patterns of thought and feeling, moves people together. The heart of Creative Music Therapy lies in the fact of musical dialogue – in 'the pattern which connects'. The case studies in this book have shown how music can make contact in sometimes extreme circumstances where words have often failed. Conversely, where words are available it makes a qualitatively different mode of communication possible. The main (yet unspoken) question the music therapist asks is simply 'Can we make music together?' From the first contact, from the first faltering notes we start to forge the 'musical between' where music is not just a physical presence between us but a creative sharing of musical thought, feeling, form and meaning. Buber's concept of 'meeting' seems the best description of this quality of relationship:

> In the most powerful moments of dialogic, where in truth 'deep calls unto deep', it becomes unmistakably clear that it is not the wand of the individual or the social, but of a third which draws the circle around the happening. On the far side of the subjective, on this side of the objective, on the narrow ridge, where I and Thou meet, there is the realm of 'between'. (Buber 1966)

Dialogue is the heart of Creative Music Therapy because communication is the heart of music. But it is communication largely relieved of representation: instead music communicates communication itself, and music therapy uses this to show that in the most unlikely circumstances communication is still possible.

ENDS AND MEANS

I began the first part of this book with the question a client put to me at a first session: 'Are we just making music?' It was a fair question, since something bearing the title 'music *therapy*' might be presumed to entail more than 'just making music'. I think I can now answer him honestly with 'yes, we are just making music', but with the qualification that though it is indeed 'all' we are doing, the implications of this fact are not as simple as they might sound. 'Just making music' covers the world of musical experience lived by the people written about in this book – from the light-hearted to the profound; the entertaining to the life-saving.

Much of the difference of opinion amongst various current approaches to music therapy centres on whether music-making is an end in itself or whether a means to other, therapeutically defined ends. The simplest example of the latter is that of 'music psychotherapy', where music-making is explicitly intended to facilitate verbal therapeutic processes. This is not, however, to say that 'just making music' is always without therapeutic aims and intentions. It is a matter of emphasis as to where the central locus of the therapy is seen to be.

At the beginning of the century the philosopher R.C. Collingwood (1938) made a distinction between 'art' and 'craft': 'according to which craft is a means to an end and must therefore be conducted according to the rules laid down by that end, whereas art is not a means but an end in itself, governed by no external purpose'. In this sense is music therapy in general, and Creative Music Therapy in particular, an art or a craft? – or is it once again a hybrid form?

I leave this as a question at this stage, though it will doubtless be clear by now where my own leaning is. If I have a theory it is that music therapy works fundamentally in the way in which music itself works, and to understand what happens in music therapy we need to look from different angles at the varieties of musical processes and musical activities within and between people.

We hope that our clients in Creative Music Therapy take away with them not just a single musical encounter but an experience of a musical and personal process – but one which took place mostly in the music itself. In the Preface to *Man the Musician* (1973) Zuckerkandl quotes the injunction which Socrates received in a dream (but acted on only in the last few days of his life): 'Make music and work at it!' This could also be an ideal motto for Creative Music Therapy. In comparison to the aims and expectations of some other approaches to music therapy Creative Music Therapy, in its focus on the purely musical experience, may perhaps seem a restriction of possibility. My answer would be that, working at this level, far from being a restriction is an access to depth: that knowing a person in the phenomenal world of music is to know them significantly, and to meet them there authentically is often to meet them deeply.

CHAPTER 27

Coda

> Even after it has given its all-inclusive answers, language still leaves some questions unanswered. In music man finds answers to those very questions. Our task is to understand the nature of the questioner on the basis of music's answers to his questions. (Victor Zuckerkandl)

'Music', wrote John Blacking, 'is like the laser in the 1960s: a solution in search of problems.' Imaginative image though this is, I wonder whether Blacking would have written this had he lived to see the growth in the possibilities and applications of music therapy in the last twenty years? Blacking's statement also echoes a favourite quotation of music therapists, attributed to Novalis: 'Every illness is a musical problem: every cure a musical solution.' It will I hope be clear that, concerning Creative Music Therapy at least, any talk of 'cure' or 'solution' must not be taken too literally. The transformations which music and a creative musical relationship can achieve are indeed real enough, but are primarily the 'solutions' of the spirit: of communication and beauty, creativity and 'liveliness'. They are also often 'solutions' only 'while the music lasts' – though this need not be a negative statement, as perhaps the case studies in this book have shown.

I have made a particular plea for a more musical understanding of music therapy, one not automatically justified by words and conceptual explanations derived from other treatment theories. Nevertheless, I turn to words in order to communicate this idea, and I also need words to ask questions about music and about music therapy. This is the nub of 'music therapist's dilemma'. Notwithstanding this I believe that words are still no part of what is essential to music and, consequently, to the music therapy process in the time of the work itself. This means that, though there are indeed many ways of going about music therapy, there *need* be no verbal component to it, or any model of explanation which is substantially outside that of the musical process itself.

We need both words and music, but we also need to know that each is a different phenomenon which can work in different ways and achieve different ends. The boundary is not a rigid one, but the distinction is none the less a necessary and real one. There are, I think, few original ideas in this book. Instead there are many old ideas and old problems raising their heads within the special context of music-making which is music therapy. In what is still after all a young profession music therapists have tended largely to get involved in thinking about the aspects and issues of the 'therapy side' of this two-faced art, largely ignoring those of the 'musical' side. These musical issues are perhaps not surprisingly no different from the age-old problems of musical aesthetics, such as: what is the nature of musical expression, creativity, beauty? Is music representational? Is musical thinking 'real' thinking? and so on. These are not irrelevant, dry academic questions but have a direct bearing on how music therapy is done, and what sense is made of it.

I have found that music therapy can give fascinating insights into why we have music in the first place: not to soothe us on the telephone or even to make us passive spectators in a concert-hall, but to forge one of the deepest and most mysterious of human meetings, which is a true connection of both heart and mind. Music therapy as a musical phenomenon raises some fascinating and necessary questions about music, about people and what happens when music and a person meet. The answers, however, are not necessarily in words.

Appendix

This book has presented one particular approach to music therapy with adult clients. Nordoff–Robbins music therapy has three centres for therapy and for training music therapists: in London, Herdecke and New York. At the time of writing only the course at Herdecke trains students substantially to work with adult clients (as opposed to children). There are plans, however, to extend the London course in 1995–6 to incorporate work with adult clients. The New York clinic teaches a module in Nordoff–Robbins therapy to students as part of a broader study of music therapy at New York University (which includes several models of practice). Readers interested in pursuing either therapy or training in this approach should, however, approach the relevant Nordoff–Robbins centre, given that the picture is likely to change in the next few years.

The Nordoff–Robbins Music Therapy Centre
2 Lissenden Gardens
London NW5 1PP

Institut für Musiktherapie
Universität Witten-Herdecke
Alfred Herrhausen Strasse 50
D-58448 Witten
Germany

Nordoff-Robbins Music Therapy Clinic
New York University
26 Washington Place
New York, NY10003
USA

For information concerning possibilities of music therapy and training in other approaches in England:

British Society for Music Therapy
25 Rosslyn Avenue
East Barnet
Hertfordshire EN4 8DH

References

Books or articles marked with an asterisk are recommended as further reading.

Adams, M. (1987) Measurement problems in applied music therapy research. *Journal of British Music Therapy 1*, 2.

*Aigen, K. (1991) The voice in the forest: a conception of music for music therapy. *Music Therapy 10*, 1.

*Aldridge, D. (1989a) A phenomenological comparison of the organisation of music and the self. *The Arts in Psychotherapy 16.*

*Aldridge, D. (1989b) Music, communication and medicine. *Journal of the Royal Society of Medicine 82*, December.

Aldridge, D. (1991) Creativity and consciousness: music therapy in intensive care. *The Arts in Psychotherapy 18.*

Aldridge, D. (1992) The needs of individual patients in clinical research. *Advances 8*, 4.

*Aldridge, D. (1993a) Music therapy research I: a review of the medical research literature within a general context of music therapy research. *The Arts in Psychotherapy 20.*

*Aldridge, D. (1993b) Music therapy research II: research methods suitable for music therapists. *The Arts in Psychotherapy 20.*

*Aldridge, D. (1993c) Artists or psychotherapists? *The Arts in Psychotherapy 20.*

Aldridge, D. and Aldridge, G. (1992) Two epistemologies: music therapy and medicine in the treatment of dementia. *The Arts in Psychotherapy 19.*

*Aldridge, D., Brandt, G and Wohler, D. (1990) Towards a common language in the arts therapies. *The Arts in Psychotherapy 17.*

Aldridge, D. and Lewith, G. (1993) Observational methods: a search for methods in an ecosystemic paradigm. In D. Aldridge and G. Lewith (eds) *Clinical Research Methodology for Complementary Therapies.* London: Hodder and Stoughton.

Ansdell, G. (1990) Limitations and potential: a report on a music therapy group for clients referred from a counselling service. *Journal of British Music Therapy 4*, 1.

Ansdell, G. (1991) Mapping the territory. *Journal of British Music Therapy 5*, 2.

*Bailey, D. (1992) *Improvisation.* London: The British Library.

Bannister, R. (1981) Personal construct theory and research methods. In P. Reason and J. Rowan (eds) *Human Inquiry: A Sourcebook of New Paradigm Research.* Chichester: John Wiley.

Bateson, G. (1980) *Mind and Nature.* London: Fontana.

Berendt, J.-E. (1988) *The Third Ear.* Shaftesbury: Element Books.

*Blacking, J. (1987) *A Commonsense View of all Music.* Cambridge: Cambridge University Press.

Bohm, D. and Peat, F.D. (1989) *Science, Order and Creativity.* London: Routledge.

Bos, A. (1989) *AIDS.* Stroud: Hawthorn Press.

*Bruscia, K. (1991) *Case Studies in Music Therapy.* Philadelphia: Barcelona Publishers.

*Buber, M. (1966) *The Way of Response.* New York: Schocken Books.

Buber, M. (1987) *I and Thou.* Edinburgh: T.& T. Clark.

*Bunt, L. (1994) *Music Therapy: An Art Beyond Words.* London: Routledge.

Carr, I. (1992) *Keith Jarrett: A Biography.* London: Paladin.

Campbell, D. (ed) (1991) *Music, Physician for Times to Come.* Wheaton, Illinois: Quest Books.

Clifton, T. (1975) Some comparisons between intuitive and scientific descriptions of music. *Journal of Music Theory 19*, 1.

Clifton, T. (1983) *Music as Heard.* New Haven: Yale University Press.

Collingwood, R.C. (1938) *The Principles of Art.* Oxford University Press.

Condon, W. and Ogston, W. (1966) Sound film analysis of normal and pathological behaviour patterns. *Journal of Nervous and Mental Disorders 14.*

*Cook, N. (1990) *Music, Imagination and Culture.* Oxford University Press.

Czikszentmihalyi, M. (1992) *Flow: The Psychology of Happiness.* London: Random Century.

Czikszentmihalyi, M. and Czikszentmihalyi, I.S. (eds) (1988) *Optimal Experience: Psychological Studies of Flow in Consciousness.* New York: Cambridge University Press.

Dahlhaus, C. (1982) *Esthetics of Music.* Cambridge: Cambridge University Press.

Dinnage, R. (1992) *The Ruffian on the Stair.* London: Penguin.

Elliott, D. (1993) Music as knowledge. In E. Jorgensen (ed) *Philosopher, Teacher, Musician.* Urbana: University of Illinois Press.

*Evans, D. and Rodger, I. (1992) *Anthroposophical Medicine.* London: Thorsons.

Forinash, M. (1993) An exploration into qualitative research in music therapy. *The Arts in Psychotherapy 20.*

Freud, S. (1951) *Introductory Lectures on Psychoanalysis Part I.* (Standard Edition Vol. 15.) London: Hogarth Press.

*Gilroy, A. and Lee, C. (eds) (1995) *Art and Music: Therapy and Research.* London: Routledge.

Grudin, R. (1990) *The Grace of Great Things.* New York: Ticknor and Fields.

Harrer, G. and Harrer, H. (1977) Music, emotion and autonomic function. In M. Critchley and R.A. Henson (eds) *Music and the Brain.* London: Heinemann.

Heyink, J. and Tymskra, T. (1993) The function of qualitative research. *Social Indicators Research 29.*

Hitchcock, D. (1987) The influence of Jung's psychology on the therapeutic use of music. *Journal of British Music Therapy 1*, 2.

Hull, J. (1991) *Touching the Rock.* London: Arrow.

John, D. (1992) Towards music psychotherapy. *Journal of British Music Therapy 6*, 1.

Jung, C.G. (1954) *The Practice of Psychotherapy.* London: Routledge.

Keenan, B. (1992) *An Evil Cradling.* London: Hutchinson.

Kerman, J. (1985) *Musicology.* London: Fontana.

Kermode, F. (1967) *The Sense of an Ending.* Oxford University Press.

*Kivy, P. (1990) *Music Alone.* Ithaca: Cornell University Press.

*Kivy, P. (1993) *The Fine Art of Repetition.* Cambridge University Press.

Korzybski, A. (1941) *Science and Sanity.* New York: Science Publications.

Langer, S. (1960) *Philosophy in a New Key.* Cambridge, MA: Harvard University Press.

Lee, C. (1992) The analysis of therapeutic improvisatory music with people living with the virus HIV and AIDS. Unpublished PhD thesis, City University, London.

Levarie, S. and Levy, E. (1983) *Musical Morphology: A Discourse and a Dictionary.* Ohio: Kent State University Press.

Lévi-Strauss, C. (1970) *The Raw and the Cooked.* London: Cape.

Lomas, P. (1987) *The Limits of Interpretation.* London: Penguin.

Maslow, A. (1976) *The Farther Reaches of Human Nature.* London: Penguin.

Neugebauer, L. (1992) Therapie als Dialog. Unpublished doctoral dissertation, Universität Witten-Herdecke, Germany.

*Nordoff, P. and Robbins, C. (1971) *Therapy in Music for Handicapped Children.* London: Gollancz.

Nordoff, P. and Robbins, C. (1977) *Creative Music Therapy.* New York: John Day.

Pavlicevic, M. (1991) Music in communication: improvisation in music therapy. Unpublished PhD thesis, University of Edinburgh.

*Pavlicevic, M. (1992) Music as therapy: revisiting the muses. *Journal of British Music Therapy 6*, 2.

*Pavlicevic, M. and Trevarthen, C. (1989) A musical assessment of psychiatric states in adults. *Psychopathology 22.*

*Payne, H. (1993) *Handbook of Inquiry in the Arts Therapies: One River, Many Currents.* London: Jessica Kingsley Publishers.

Popper, K. (1976) *Unended Quest.* London: Fontana.

Priestley, M. (1983) *The Herdecke Analytical Music Therapy Lectures.* Stuttgart: Klett-Cotta.

Priestley, M. (1988) Music and the Listeners. *Journal of British Music Therapy 2*, 2.

Reason, P. and Rowan, J. (1981) *Human Inquiry: A Sourcebook of New Paradigm Research.* Chichester: John Wiley.

*Rooley, A. (1990) *Performance.* Shaftesbury: Element Books.

*Ruud, E. (1980) *Music Therapy and its Relationship to Current Treatment Theories.* St Louis: Magnamusic-Baton.

Ryle, G. (1971) Knowing how and knowing that. In G.Ryle *Collected Papers.* London: Hutchinson.

*Sacks,O. (1985) *The Man who Mistook his Wife for a Hat.* London: Duckworth.

*Sacks,O. (1986) *A Leg to Stand On.* London: Pan.

*Sacks,O. (1990) Neurology and the soul *The New York Review of Books* 22.

*Sacks,O. (1991) *Awakenings.* London: Pan (revised edition).

Sacks,O. (1993) quoted in: *Bulletin of the Beth Abraham Hospital.*

Schenker, H. (1956, tr.1979) *Free Composition.* London: Faber.

*Scruton, R. (1983) *The Aesthetic Understanding.* London: Methuen.

Skille, O., Wigram, T. and Weekes, L. (1989) Vibroacoustic therapy: the effect of low frequency sound on specific physical disorders and disabilities. *Journal of British Music Therapy 3*, 2.

*Sontag, S. (1966) *Against Interpretation.* London: Vintage.

*Steiner, G. (1989) *Real Presences.* London: Faber.

Stern, D. (1985) *The Interpersonal World of the Infant:A View from Psychoanalysis and Developmental Psychology.* New York: Basic Books.

Stevens, A. (1991) *On Jung.* London: Penguin.

*Storr, A. (1976) *The Dynamics of Creation.* London: Penguin.

*Storr, A. (1988) *The School of Genius.* London: André Deutsch.

*Storr, A. (1992) *Music and the Mind.* London: Harper Collins.

Stravinsky, I. (1947) *Poetics of Music.* New York: Vintage.

Styron, W. (1992) *Darkness Visible.* London: Pan.

*Sudnow, D. (1978) *Ways of the Hand: The Organization of Improvised Conduct.* Cambridge, MA: MIT Press.

*Thomson, M. (1989) *On Art and Therapy.* London: Virago.

Todes, C. (1990) *Shadow over my Brain.* Gloucestershire: Windrush Press.

Towse, E. (1991) Relationships in music therapy: do music therapy techniques discourage the emergence of transference? *British Journal of Psychotherapy 74,* 4.

*Winnicott, D.W. (1991) *Playing and Reality.* London: Tavistock-Routledge.

Zohar, D. (1990) *The Quantum Self.* London: Bloomsbury.

*Zuckerkandl, V. (1956) *Sound and Symbol: Music and the External World.* New Jersey: Princeton University Press.

*Zuckerkandl, V. (1959) *The Sense of Music.* New Jersey: Princeton University Press.

*Zuckerkandl, V. (1973) *Man the Musician.* New Jersey: Princeton University Press.

Subject Index

References in italic indicate figures or tables.

Author Index

A Note on the Compact disk

The compact disc which accompanies this book contains extracts from the music therapy sessions of clients written about in the case studies. These are designed both to illustrate points being made in the text and also to convey impressions which are not possible in words. Though many of the excerpts are short and need the text to put them in context, a few longer examples are included which stand on their own as improvisations. The reader is advised to listen to the CD in conjunction with reading a particular case. A CD track and its number is indicated by the legend [⊙1] in the text. At the end of each case study is a 'Listening Guide', again with the track numbers and with a short text to give necessary information about the excerpt (who plays what, the context of the excerpt, etc.).

Unfortunately the recording quality of the material is far from even – the source tapes ranging from fifteen-year-old reel-to-reel to modern DAT recordings. Also the acoustic where the sessions took place varies as widely: from the luxury of a purpose-built music therapy studio to the converted broom cupboard which many music therapists will no doubt recognise. Whilst all this does not make for easy listening it does convey both the realities of the music therapist's daily existence and, I think, adds an individual atmosphere to each of the cases as they are heard.

Compact disc Tracks

[1]	Emanuella
[2]	Emanuella
[3]	Emanuella
[4]	Emanuella
[5]	Emanuella
[6]	Just a Minute...
[7]	Herr G.
[8]	Karl
[9]	Karl
[10]	Herr Putz
[11]	Herr Putz
[12]	David
[13]	David
[14]	David
[15]	David
[16]	Charlie
[17]	Jack
[18]	Jack
[19]	The Wednesday Group
[20]	Gisela
[21]	Jane
[22]	Jane